QIGONG
illustrated

Christina J. Barea

Human Kinetics

Library of Congress Cataloging-in-Publication Data

Barea, Christina J.
  Qigong illustrated / Christina J. Barea.
    p. cm.
  ISBN-13: 978-0-7360-8981-4 (softcover)
  ISBN-10: 0-7360-8981-0 (softcover)
  1. Qi gong. 2. Qi gong--Pictorial works. I. Title.
  RA781.8.B37 2011
  613.7'1489--dc22

                              2010028589

ISBN-10: 0-7360-8981-0 (print)
ISBN-13: 978-0-7360-8981-4 (print)

This publication is written and published to provide accurate and authoritative information relevant to the subject matter presented. It is published and sold with the understanding that the author and publisher are not engaged in rendering legal, medical, or other professional services by reason of their authorship or publication of this work. If medical or other expert assistance is required, the services of a competent professional person should be sought.

The Web addresses cited in this text were current as of August 2010, unless otherwise noted.

Acquisitions Editor: Tom Heine; **Developmental Editor:** Laura Floch; **Assistant Editor:** Elizabeth Evans; **Copyeditor:** Alisha Jeddeloh; **Graphic Designer:** Bob Reuther; **Graphic Artist:** Tara Welsch; **Cover Designer:** Keith Blomberg; **Photographer (cover):** Neil Bernstein; **Photographer (interior):** Benjamin Lapid; **Photo Asset Manager:** Laura Fitch; **Visual Production Assistant:** Joyce Brumfield; **Photo Production Manager:** Jason Allen; **Art Manager:** Kelly Hendren; **Associate Art Manager:** Alan L. Wilborn; **Printer:** United Graphics

We thank Studio B in Decatur, Georgia, for assistance in providing the location for the photo shoot for this book.

Human Kinetics books are available at special discounts for bulk purchase. Special editions or book excerpts can also be created to specification. For details, contact the Special Sales Manager at Human Kinetics.

Printed in the United States of America   10 9 8 7 6 5 4 3 2 1

The paper in this book is certified under a sustainable forestry program.

Human Kinetics
Web site: www.HumanKinetics.com

United States: Human Kinetics
P.O. Box 5076
Champaign, IL 61825-5076
800-747-4457
e-mail: humank@hkusa.com

Canada: Human Kinetics
475 Devonshire Road Unit 100
Windsor, ON N8Y 2L5
800-465-7301 (in Canada only)
e-mail: info@hkcanada.com

Europe: Human Kinetics
107 Bradford Road
Stanningley
Leeds LS28 6AT, United Kingdom
+44 (0) 113 255 5665
e-mail: hk@hkeurope.com

Australia: Human Kinetics
57A Price Avenue
Lower Mitcham, South Australia 5062
08 8372 0999
e-mail: info@hkaustralia.com

New Zealand: Human Kinetics
P.O. Box 80
Torrens Park, South Australia 5062
0800 222 062
e-mail: info@hknewzealand.com

                                                                    E5029

QIGONG
illustrated

For Matteo
Keep your Heart chakra open

Contents

Foreword

Today more than ever, it is imperative that we take responsibility for our health and well-being. As a society, we have allowed ourselves to become dependent on someone else or something else to fix our ailments, our bodies, our lives. Although these repairs can accomplish many things, too often they are not complete or not permanent.

When we realize that we are not a group of disparate systems (physical, mental, emotional, spiritual) but integrated beings, we discover the secret to making health care really work. Qigong is one such system that provides for our whole being. It is an ancient form of exercise and meditation that has brought many people into true mental and physical health. It is a mind–body practice that integrates postures, movement, breathing techniques, and focused intention.

Although qigong has been used in China for thousands of years, few people in the West have heard of it until recently. Over the past decade the National Institutes of Health (NIH) and other organizations have conducted research that validates what is commonly accepted in China and have made those research findings applicable to Western culture.

As we turn to ancient forms of health practice, it is important that we have a knowledgeable guide. Christina brings us a simple method of achieving a state of wellness. She draws on the roots of Chinese medical theory, allowing the theory to come alive into a personal practice. You will have the opportunity to discover the energetics behind the theory firsthand.

Christina's background and training are suitable to the subject of complementary and alternative health modalities as she combines her personal experience with ancient wisdom. I have had the fortune of seeing Christina in many settings: as a student, a practitioner, and a teacher. As a student, she demonstrated the willingness to be open and the discipline to practice. As a practitioner, she is compassionate and able to assist patients in profound ways. As a teacher, she speaks to our minds while speaking to our hearts.

Christina's writing style matches her teaching style: simple, direct, thorough. She makes the information accessible, stimulates our interest, and reassures us that we can accomplish these exercises and achieve the desired results. Christina uses ancient terms but brings them into current usage, and she includes the right amount of information to acquaint us with the concepts. The detailed illustrations enhance our understanding of the concepts.

Qigong Illustrated is your guide to achieving health and well-being with gentle effectiveness.

Dr. Bernard Shannon, DMQ (China)
Executive director, International Institute of Medical Qigong

Preface

Approaching qigong for the first time can feel challenging, especially if you are reading classics written by enlightened masters or watching videos of experts relying on almost a lifetime of practice in their art. It's easy to get lost in the mystical concepts of Heaven, Earth, jing, qi, and shen or confused with Chinese language and traditional Chinese medicine (TCM) theory. However, the truth is that even we mortals have a chance at excellent health and longevity without having to go swimming too deeply in the river of knowledge. Practicing qigong doesn't require changing religions, speaking Chinese, or even having a strong, supple body. The beauty of qigong lies within the simplicity of its meaning—the practice of energy (breathing) cultivation over time. To practice qigong, all you have to do is take a deep breath and begin.

Qigong is enjoying a revival around the world, attracting people interested in its healing power, its graceful motions, and its incredible physical feats. It has been credited with curing diseases where Western medicine has failed and is now being prescribed by respected physicians at notable hospitals such as Stanford in California. The slow moves of qigong are attracting men, women, children, and seniors, granting them vibrant health, vitality, and longevity. And its demonstrations of incredible physical strength or prowess, such as by traveling Shaolin monks, fill auditoriums. This rise in qigong's popularity and its various applications accentuates the need for clear and accurate information. Although an ever-growing number of texts and teachers are becoming available in English, the bulk remains in Chinese, contributing to the dissemination of misinformation and widespread ambiguity.

The purpose of this book is to provide a solid foundation with which to begin building a quality qigong practice you can continue for years to come. Within these pages you will find clear definitions that demystify the elusive concepts of qi and cultivation as well as a step-by-step approach to qigong with easy-to-follow instructions for even the most inexperienced practitioner. The content of this book is the result of the knowledge and skills passed on to me by excellent teachers, along with the experience gained teaching in a variety of venues. My goal is to pass on the best information possible to make sure your qigong practice is both effective and enjoyable.

Most students are attracted to qigong because of the apparent simplicity of the moves, and they enjoy the rush of energy once they begin. Yet, in all classes core concepts and questions consistently surface. Does qi really exist, and how can I identify it? I have injuries or surgeries, so how can I practice qigong? Can qigong heal me? This book answers these fundamental questions and highlights the major principles of qigong that will ensure that your practice is safe, enjoyable, and true to the art.

After you finish this book, you will be able to integrate your qigong knowledge seamlessly into other qigong styles or even martial arts such as tai chi chuan (the fighting application of tai chi) or kung fu, making everything contained in these pages practical for more than just qigong. You may, of course, decide to keep it simple and not explore any further, but be assured that within these pages lies enough material for at least three years of solid practice that will always reveal something new.

The first section of this book includes chapters 1 through 4, which address the most fundamental aspects of qigong, such as the definition of *qi* and *gong* as individual words as well as *qigong* as an entire concept. Chapters 2, 3, and 4 introduce the practitioner to the Three Treasures, commonly known in China as jing, qi, and shen but simplified here as posture, breath, and intention, providing a clear idea of what practicing qigong involves. Each chapter builds on the others, providing a flowing description of this multifaceted concept.

The rest of the book guides you through a complete qigong practice, from an opening sequence to cooling down and meditation. Each qigong exercise gives clear instructions on movements, breathing patterns, and visualizations. The Daoist Five and Eight Silk Brocade are core routines and have symbolic references to the Five Elements and eight animals.

Throughout the book you will find special elements—sidebars and FAQs—that include tips for improving your practice and answers to the most common questions asked by beginning practitioners. The information they contain is as important as the exercises themselves.

Note About Chinese Terminology

Throughout the book you might notice that some words are capitalized. TCM uses words that sound similar to Western anatomical terminology. However, when TCM uses certain words (identified by a capital initial letter), it implies an expanded meaning of the body part. For example, *heart* is the Western term and refers to the heart organ and its physiological functions when it is not capitalized, whereas *Heart* (TCM) refers to both the heart organ and its energetic and spiritual functions and representations, including its definition and correspondences according to the Five Elements theory, which you will learn about in this book.

It is truly my pleasure to put knowledge, experience, and passion together for your benefit as you begin this journey toward self-discovery and sustainable good health. I firmly believe that there are no accidents or coincidences; therefore, this book arrives at the perfect time. As you turn the pages, remember to breathe, wiggle your toes, and enjoy the journey of qigong. I send you many blessings for great health.

Acknowledgments

My journey through qigong, Daoism, and martial arts is blessed with the presence of great friends and teachers. Although they may have entered my life through one door or the other, today I see no separation. Teachers are friends who care enough to show you the path, and friends are teachers who through their unfailing loyalty show you unconditional love and compassion. Undoubtedly they are the people who have molded my decisions and led me to the place I am today.

To the following people I extend my deepest gratitude; without your influence, guidance, and help I would not be the person I am today, nor would the creation of this book have been possible.

To my teachers Sifu Jerry Alan Johnson, Sifu Bernard Shannon, and Sifu Florin Szondi, my deepest gratitude for sharing your knowledge, experience, and lessons, in addition to allowing me to be part of your lives as a friend.

To Sheri Gilburth and Essud Fungcap, thank you for being such gracious friends and giving your time to be models. I look forward to continuing on this path together!

Thank you to Benjamin Lapid for the photos, Laura Floch for editing, Joe Rodgers for the concept, Tom Heine for the follow-through, J.D. Scott for the studio, and the entire staff of Human Kinetics for the completion of the project.

To Christopher MacDonald, I am grateful for your support while this book was created. Your love, generosity, and words of Light were a blessing. Aho!

Thank you to my two best friends and true angels walking on earth: Lourdes Gonzalez and Victoria Cannon.

To my family: Matteo Aramis, my son, thank you for your unconditional love and patience, and thanks to JoAnne Harris (Mom), Julio Barea (Dad), Julio Barea III, Phillip Barea, Betty Harris (Mama), Pilar Barea, and Diego Barea for being there throughout all my many changes.

And in remembrance of my ancestors and departed friends who have inspired me in so many ways: Carmen Barea Bosch (Cachi), Julio Barea (Papa), James Harris (Granddaddy), Father Federico Consla (Spike), Edwin del Toro, and Jose Ignacio Bartolomei.

Chapter 1

Art and Practice of Qigong

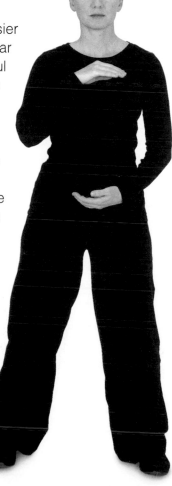

Qigong is a beautiful art with so many facets that it's easier to describe it as a spherical concept rather than a linear progression of ideas. The image of a sphere is also useful to describe how qigong can become a complete lifestyle rather than an isolated practice. As we begin exploring the sphere of qigong, bring your awareness to how it already may be a part of your life and allow the deeper understanding of its purpose and method to extend into new areas.

Let's begin our journey by envisioning a large bubble with the word *qigong* inside it, floating in front of you. Can you see the letters? Are they black? Fuzzy? Sharp? Is the word legible from left to right, or is it upside down? How it actually appears doesn't matter; just hold the word *qigong* in front of you. Inside the bubble, you can see that there is also space, or air, or atmosphere completely surrounding these floating letters. Now envision that you could arrive toward the letters of qigong from any angle. It could be from left, right, front, back, above, below, sideways, diagonal, and so on, multiplied over and over by the infinite angles contained within a sphere. Each angle will change the perspective or appearance of the letters, and this is exactly how to define qigong. It depends on how you approach it!

How do you pronounce qigong?

Qi is pronounced "chee," as in "cheese." *Gong* is pronounced "goong," as in "gooey," but with an "-ng" at the end. Although it is commonly pronounced "gong," as in the large cymbal struck with a mallet, that pronunciation is not quite accurate. The word *qigong* is actually two words in Chinese: *qi* and *gong*. It is common to write two words that go together without a space in between, and therefore we use the term *qigong*. It is also correct to write *QiGong* as a title.

The art and practice of qigong is complex and encompasses countless meditations, exercises, breathing techniques, life habits, healing modalities, treatment protocols, spiritual beliefs, and more. It includes feng shui, Chinese astrology, medical qigong therapy, and Daoist practices, to name a few, each one applying the principles of qigong in a different way. But the richness of the practice should only entice one to continue its deep exploration. It would be unrealistic to expect to master the sphere of qigong in just a few lessons. One needs patience, persistence, and flexibility, thereby leading to the following definition of qigong: the practice of energy cultivation over time.

Defining Qigong

As we just mentioned, the word *qigong* is simply translated as "the practice of energy cultivation over time;" however, the word holds a much deeper meaning. Chinese is a descriptive language where each character represents a three-dimensional concept, so *qigong* stands for a wealth of ideas and practices, as we are about to discover. Let's begin by breaking down the word *qigong* into two smaller components, *qi* and *gong*. (See figure 1.1 to see *qi* and *gong* in Chinese characters.)

氣
功

Figure 1.1 Chinese characters for *qi* and *gong*.

Qi has several translations, including "energy," "life-force," "breath," "air," "mist," "steam," and more. But simply stated, it's the particular *energy* of an object. It is believed that all objects have energy, including people, animals, plants—in short, anything contained on the Earth and in the Heavens. Perhaps you've heard about this energy and are wondering, "Well, what does *energy* mean?" You might even be a skeptic who doesn't believe that qi exists. Defining energy can seem like asking someone to believe in a mystical force that permeates the universe and all living beings. And yet, that's true—it is and it does.

Qi is mystical in the sense that we don't fully comprehend how to define it, control it, or measure it. It exists, yet it constantly reveals new layers of discovery. The limitation of our understanding of those things we cannot see, feel, or hear is the same limitation we have in understanding the power of qi. But let's find a more practical and perhaps scientific approach to defining qi.

Metaphor of the Three Treasures

The collective qi of the universe can be divided into three realms according to the quality of the energy. Each of these realms has unique characteristics that distinguish it from the others. Because each realm is an important part of the interaction of all energy, it is called a *treasure*. The relationship between the three realms, or *the Three Treasures*, becomes a metaphor for three-tiered interactions, many of which we will learn about in this book (see table 1.1).

TABLE 1.1

The Three Treasures

Lower treasure	Middle treasure	Upper treasure
Physical	Emotional	Mental
Earth	Man	Heaven
Body	Breath	Mind
Martial	Medical	Spiritual
Jing	Qi	Shen
Lower dantian	Middle dantian	Upper dantian
1st wei qi field	2nd wei qi field	3rd wei qi field

A basic way of defining qi is through the five energies of cells: heat, light, sound, magnetic, and electric. Simply stated, each cell emits wavelengths of heat, light, sound, magnetism, and electricity. Each of those wavelengths can be measured, altered, and controlled. We know that some of those wavelengths can be perceived without the aid of special devices. We see a wide gamma of light, but we can't see X rays or infrared radiation. Does that mean they don't exist? Absolutely not—they do exist. We can hear a car engine running, birds chirping, and music being played at the symphony, but we can't hear the sound of a dog whistle. Does that mean it doesn't exist? Just whistle at Fido—he will answer! Qi is this type of energy but not just each one in isolation; it's all of them put together. Together, these energies

Is qigong a religion? Is it the same as Falun Gong?

No. Qigong is not related to a religion or faith of any kind. The basis of qigong is working with universal energy. The foundation of qigong is that it exists everywhere independent from language, faith, gender, nationality, or race. The physical and energetic movements taught to Falun Gong practitioners are considered qigong. But, although Falun Gong claims to be independent of political, social, and religious ideals, its moral and ethical requirements have generated controversy in mainland China, where it is perceived as a threat to the stability of the Chinese Communist Party.

give a living cell a multidimensional quality that includes function, communication, and connection well beyond the boundaries of the physical realm.

Let's quickly examine a phrase that often accompanies popular definitions of qi and qigong: "Everything is connected." Many people wonder how we all can be connected when, for example, there are thousands of miles between millions of people in this world. Well, let's go back to the five energies of cells. We established that each one of those energies emits a wavelength, right? That wavelength travels as far as the intensity of the emitter. Visualize a magnet. It emits a field around it that is proportional to its strength—the stronger the magnet, the bigger the field. Humans are the same. We are a huge magnet or battery emitting a field of invisible, inaudible, and otherwise insensible wavelengths from our bodies. Qigong masters have learned how to feel, emit, intensify, diminish, and otherwise control the field by controlling their bodies. It's easy to imagine that learning how to do this would require a lot of practice—in other words, gong.

Gong refers to practice which leads to "merit" or "achievement." Saying "qigong" implies practicing qi cultivation over time. The question now becomes, "How do I learn to cultivate qi?" Ah, well, that's the hard part. Actually, it's not hard; it just requires patience, practice, and discipline. Like any sport, art, or skill, qigong must be developed. One needs to begin to absorb the many nuances of the skill before being able to produce something that is both beautiful and powerful. However, there is infinite joy in taking time to learn an art of any kind. The learning process reveals our strengths, talents, and inspiration and patiently waits for us to work with our weaknesses.

Naturally, if one's objective is to be able to do magic with qigong, then the *gong* part of training will be more difficult and take much longer before results are seen. Fortunately, when practicing qigong for health, we can begin to see results immediately. Just a little guidance can get you started on the fast track to a great qigong practice.

Three Applications of Qigong

There are several ways to practice qigong, and the approach taken begins to define which type of qigong you'll be doing and perhaps the difficulty of obtaining results. Qigong practices can generally be classified into three applications: martial, medical, and spiritual. Each of these applications relies on the same foundations and definition of qigong but with a much different intention. Knowing that the foundation of qigong is the same regardless of the application is important because it explains why a person can practice one type of qigong yet obtain benefits in other areas.

To better understand the differences between each application, we can begin by asking, "Why? Why are you practicing this qigong?" The answer to this question is fundamental since it reveals the first path that you'll travel upon to discover the sphere of qigong. Ultimately, if your practice is long enough, you'll have the answer to all perspectives. But for now, let's assume you are interested in the health benefits.

Keep in mind that many qigong movements may look identical to the observer but are a completely different exercise to the practitioner. This is referred to as changing the *intention* of the qigong. We'll return to intention shortly. First, let's take a quick look at the three applications of qigong.

Martial

Qigong is not solely a martial art, although there are aspects of qigong training that can be and are used in martial arts training. Martial qigong means practicing qigong in order to develop fighting skill or physical aptitude. It focuses on the body and increasing strength, resistance, and power. Training with qigong for martial purposes emphasizes tendons, muscles, and bones. The various types of Iron training are martial qigong (e.g., Iron Palm, Iron Shirt, Iron Fist). Martial artists bending spears with their necks or breaking seemingly impenetrable objects demonstrate this type of qigong.

Medical

Medical qigong means practicing qigong with the intention of improving one's health and wellness. It focuses on qi

What are common side effects of practicing qigong?

Qigong stimulates the flow of energy, creating tangible expressions of it's movement. Because of each person's individuality, how it feels may not always be the same; however, some common descriptions are tingling, buzzing, raised energy level, nausea, dizziness, diarrhea, insomnia, deep sleep, hot, cold, rushing wind, sharp pains, dull pains, etc. These are all indications that qi is moving and readjusting. In all cases, these symptoms should pass within a very short time (less than an hour). If, for any reason, you have symptoms that last more than an hour, contact your qualified qigong instructor for guidance.

Can I practice qigong if I have an injury?

Maybe—it depends on the injury. Some factors to consider are location, depth (skin versus internal organ), severity (pulled muscle versus severed tendons), and date of incident (fresh versus old). A good guideline would be that fresh wounds or injuries need time to heal. If the majority of the healing is done, then it may be safe for you to begin a qigong practice. If you will be learning from this book and without a teacher, please contact a qualified qigong instructor or your physician for specific guidance.

Qigong for Health

The purpose of this book is to provide instruction on qigong exercises that will improve health. Qigong is gaining popularity around the world for its ability to provide profound healing to people with a wide range of medical conditions. Well-respected medical doctors are prescribing qigong for people with hypertension (high blood pressure), arthritis, attention deficit/hyperactivity disorder (ADHD), and osteoporosis, as well as for those who are undergoing cancer therapies. Major hospitals such as Stanford in Palo Alto, California, have included qigong classes on campus in order to provide group and individual instruction to patients. Qigong provides relief from symptoms of these and many other conditions without the use of medication and without the unwanted side effects. As more scientific research concludes with significant positive results, the West will continue to turn its eye to the East, searching for answers in the wisdom passed down for thousands of years.

The benefits of qigong extend far beyond relief from medical conditions. Anyone can benefit from this gentle art. Because qigong works on three levels simultaneously, it strengthens the entire body, including organs, tissues, bones, blood, and mind, becoming a powerful tool for prevention. Qigong provides benefits in the following health areas:

- ► Increased blood circulation and oxygenation
- ► Regulation of blood pressure
- ► Increased heart strength
- ► Increased lung strength and capacity
- ► Increased resilience of tendons and ligaments
- ► Increased immune function
- ► Balancing of hormones and endocrine system
- ► Increased bone mass

- ► Increased overall energy
- ► Increased flexibility
- ► Increased balance
- ► Increased coordination
- ► Increased focus and attention
- ► Increased ability to relax
- ► Stress relief

Qigong is being practiced by millions of people around the world as complementary therapy for the following conditions and more:

- ► Cancer
- ► Fibromyalgia
- ► Asthma
- ► Chronic fatigue syndrome
- ► Heart disease
- ► High blood pressure
- ► Low blood pressure

- ► Thyroid conditions
- ► Stress management
- ► Arthritis
- ► Recovery from surgery
- ► Recovery from injuries
- ► Diabetes
- ► ADHD

Qigong offers a wealth of benefits regardless of which application one chooses to practice. As we go forward, our focus will be on qigong for health. All the information presented can be beneficial for a wide range of health conditions. But even just regular practice of qigong can be great for prevention. Qigong for health is easy to learn and doesn't require lifting heavy weights or twisting in odd positions, greatly reducing the risk of exercise-induced injuries. With the guidance of a qualified instructor, qigong can be tailored to suit your particular needs and health condition, making it an enjoyable practice that will last a lifetime.

circulation and target areas for body mind conditioning. It also tends to be gentler than martial qigong. Training with medical qigong places focus on joint flexibility, cardiorespiratory capacity, organ health, and blood circulation. Noncompetitive tai chi (or taiji) is an example of this. We will be focusing on qigong for health in this book.

Spiritual

Spiritual qigong means practicing qigong for the purpose of developing one's spiritual path. It focuses on developing, refining, and strengthening one's spirit. It tends to be more on the mental side as opposed to physical and can be the most gentle form of qigong (but not the easiest!). It is sometimes referred to as *shen gong*. Meditations and prayer are examples of this qigong.

People who are interested in developing aptitude in just one of the three applications of qigong are often pleased to discover that as they improve in one area, improvement is also found in another—so much so that it is often subject of debate among qigong instructors whether one can really separate qigong into categories. I believe that at an introductory level, they can be separated and that certain exercises are intended for specific applications, but if one practices long enough, the applications begin to blend and are strengthened simultaneously. This idea leads us back to the example of the qigong sphere, demonstrating again that the practice of qigong can be more of an integrative lifestyle rather than an isolated practice.

In addition to the three applications of qigong as described previously (martial, medical, spiritual), there is another category of qigong called "medical qigong therapy." This type of qigong is one of the four branches of Traditional Chinese Medicine and is a healing modality where qi is emitted from a therapist to a patient for the purpose of improving their health. It is different from the previous definition of qigong in that this category includes the methods, protocols, and treatments particular to qi emission therapy.

Can anyone practice qigong?

Yes! Anyone can start qigong at just about any time—including seniors and children, women, and men of all ages. However, depending on your particular body condition, it may be necessary to adapt certain movements. Most of these qigong movements can also be practiced from a chair. Just focus on following the directions for body from the waist up, keeping the bottom half of the body stationary. Integrate the directions for breath and mind as directed.

Medical qigong therapy is often referred to with different names such as "Chinese energetic medicine," "qi emission therapy," "acupuncture without needles," and even "medical qigong." Although it's somewhat confusing, the key difference is in the action of emitting qi from one person to another for the purpose of healing. Note that qigong as defined in this book is also part of Medical qigong therapy in that a therapist would recommend these qigong exercises as part of the patients "at home" or "self-healing" process.

Three Components of Qigong

Qigong as a concept implies the union of three components: body, breath, and mind. These three components *combined* are what separate qigong from just plain exercise. Regular exercise of any variety usually works with breath and body. When lifting weights, most people would probably only focus on keeping the body in alignment and remembering to breathe while performing each repetition. Aerobics works the same way—repeat the movement and breathe when you can. It works, but it's not qigong. For qigong to be effective, we must integrate our mind into the practice. So, if we are doing a qigong move but not paying attention to breath, then it's not qigong. Or, if we are doing something that looks like qigong, and we're breathing at the right time but our mind is on our grocery list or the chores we have to do after class, then again, it's not qigong. Qigong is deceptively simple. After all, it looks so easy: blissful face, gentle motions, no sweating. No problem, right? Not exactly. It's the consciousness, deliberation, and visualization, or *intention*, that we add to the movements that makes the difference.

The following states the concept of these three components in an easy-to-remember equation:

Posture + breath + intention = qigong.

A good qigong form works on all three components simultaneously. At the beginning, while learning how to move the body according to the routine, the focus is mostly on the body or posture. When one has committed the flow to memory, then the focus can shift to breathing at the right time. Finally, once the body and the breath are working in harmony, then one can move on to the mind, or intention, of the exercise. The best qigong, the one that provides great healing, is the qigong that incorporates all three levels in a coordinated flow with a clear purpose. This is the qigong that reveals layers and layers of discovery. In the next three chapters we will look at these components separately and learn how to integrate them into a powerful qigong practice.

Qigong for health is more than just doing exercises that feel good. It's an internal strengthening workout that provides real and measurable results. As qi moves through the body, it clears away old charges that may no longer serve your highest good and establishes new patterns that lead to better physical, emotional, and mental health. Qigong is an excellent way to develop increased cardiorespiratory capacity, tendon and ligament strength and resilience, balance, stamina, and strength. Over time, a thorough qigong practice can provide profound long-term changes to your entire body-mind composition, returning you to the driver seat of your health and life, ending a cycle of reaction and entering a cycle of creation.

Selecting a Qigong Instructor

So you're ready to begin practicing qigong with an instructor? Great! There are a few guidelines to keep in mind when beginning the search. First, qigong is an unregulated practice, which means that there can be significant differences in knowledge and teaching style between instructors; therefore, you should be prepared to ask many questions before jumping into a class. Some key qualities to look for in an instructor are as follows:

- ▶ *Experience*. How many years has the instructor been teaching? Is her knowledge base inclusive of multiple styles, or does she teach just one?
- ▶ *Ability to adapt*. Can the instructor tailor a class to accommodate your specific needs? A good instructor should be able to fit just about anyone into a qigong class and adapt the movements for people with injuries or other physical conditions.
- ▶ *Commitment*. What level of commitment is the instructor requesting from you as the student? Beware of excessively high prices and pressure to commit to long time frames.
- ▶ *Attitude*. Find an instructor with whom you feel comfortable. Beware of instructors who are consistently dismissive of your questions or who tend to insult other schools and teachers.

Be sure to do your research! There are a couple of reputable organizations that certify qigong instructors. Try contacting the National Qigong Association (www .nqa.org) or the International Institute of Medical Qigong (www.medicalqigong.org).

Chapter 2

Posture

The first step to achieving an effective qigong practice is noticing your posture and then correcting the alignment of your joints before beginning movement. This chapter is dedicated to creating a solid foundation on which to build your qigong practice to gain the greatest benefit and avoid injury.

This level of defining qigong, *posture*, relates to the first level of the Three Treasures of our being—jing, or essence (see page 3 in chapter 1 for more on the Three Treasures). At our most tangible level, we manifest this essence in the quality of our bones, tissues, muscles, and overall vitality. Traditional Chinese medicine (TCM) teaches that when the jing is depleted, overall health is compromised. Jing deficiency is often at the root of many conditions that display symptoms of lethargy, weakness, frailty, and infertility. The body's jing is consumed daily through various activities and lifestyle choices, but if we pay attention to healthy eating habits and don't physically overexert ourselves, then the probability of developing a jing deficiency is reduced. In addition, a person with healthy jing is able to convert it to energy (qi) and radiate a healthy glow.

What type of clothing should I wear while practicing qigong?

Because qigong is a practice in moving energy both internally and externally, it is recommended that you wear clothing that facilitates that movement. Therefore, select loose-fitting pants and shirts that don't squeeze any part of the body, and wear natural fibers such as cotton in the summer and silk in the winter. Long sleeves and pants and mandarin collars are traditionally worn because they help to keep the extremities warm and keep the qi close to the skin. Wear gym shoes for stability.

For those not familiar with TCM, jing can be difficult to understand. But if we think of it as the substance that gives power, life, and strength to our body, it is easier to understand. For example, visualize an arm and think of all the bones, tissues, muscles, blood, lymph, and so on that form it. Independent of the specific arm you visualized, these are the essential components. Now, visualize that arm on a single person in three situations: (1) on a person who has not eaten in three days but is otherwise healthy, (2) on a person who consistently eats a diet of junk food and lives a reckless lifestyle of overindulgences in drugs and sexual activity, and (3) on a person who eats well and practices moderation.

In each of these situations, the person will have the same overall constitution of bones and tissues but will have a very different quality of jing. In the first situation, the jing will be low and the person will be weak and unable to exert strength in the arm for more than a few instances. The lack of strength is from low jing due to lack of nutrition because food is an important factor in determining the quality of a person's jing. However, this person will recover quickly upon resuming regular meals. In the second situation, the jing will be low due to poor diet and overindulgences, and the capacity to exert strength for a long period of time will be compromised. The jing in this case will need more time to replenish and return to a normal level. However, if sustained for too long as a chronic deficiency, the low level of jing could lead to irreparable damage. In the third situation, the jing remains at a constant level, enabling the person to properly exert strength in the arm according to his physical constitution. Therefore, jing is demonstrated as the subtle yet definitive substance that gives life, strength, and vitality to the body.

As we just mentioned, there are several factors which contribute to the quality of a person's jing. These factors include: genetic predisposition, congenital constitution, dietary patterns and preferences, lifestyle choices such as activity (including sexual activity) and rest, and the use of supplements, stimulants, and drugs both prescription and recreational. Because each person has a unique balance between these factors, it is challenging to generalize about which is the best way to improve each person's health. For some people increasing jing may mean getting more sleep and rest, and for others it may mean significantly improving their diet. In any case, paying close attention to your particular external and internal choices will provide valuable insight on how to maintain or improve your jing. It is safe to say that you don't want to waste jing. Jing is something that deserves to be conserved and used carefully. After all, the more jing we have, the more strength and longevity we enjoy.

Jing also relates to the Kidneys in the Five Elements (which we will discuss in more detail in Chapter 4). Remember from the preface that the TCM definition of Kidneys involves more than just the actual organs and includes its energetic and spiritual components. In this regard, the Kidneys are said to store the jing making them the battery, or powerhouse, of the body. So if the Kidneys are strong and vital, then our overall vitality is also strong. The quickest way to rebuild the Kidneys and replenish jing is by eating foods that nourish the Water element. These include, but are not limited to, stews like Ox Tail Soup or Lamb Stew both prepared including the bones, black beans, spinach and other deep green leaves, micro-greens like wheatgrass juice and spirulina, and certain salty foods like seaweed.

Correct Postural Alignment

Correct posture refers to the alignment of the bones in relation to the joints for the purpose of maximizing qi flow and minimizing obstructions. In qigong therapy, it is said that wherever qi does not flow, disease sets in. Qi is carried in the Blood like water in a river and flows throughout every part of our body. If there are sharp bends in the river, qi slows down; if the river straightens, there is less resistance and the flow increases. By paying attention to how our bones are stacked on top of each other, we can minimize the number of bends in the body and thereby facilitate free-flowing qi.

Free-flowing qi is important on two levels. First, it washes through the body and cleanses the organs, fasciae, and blood. Blood carries qi along with oxygen and nutrients, and therefore it makes sense that wherever Blood is circulating, healing is occurring or disease is not setting in. Qi movement in this case means that there is no holding onto stressors of any kind and that health and relaxation are actively supported. Qigong therapy recognizes that external influences, including physical, emotional, spiritual, and mental influences, have a real energetic charge that can be associated with specific parts of the body. That is the foundation of the Five Elements theory, which we will discuss in chapter 4.

One important reason for maintaining correct alignment of the body during qigong practice is that it keeps the major

When and how often should I practice qigong?

Qigong is best practiced early in the morning when the circulating energy can boost your stamina for the rest of the day. Qigong practice should never begin late in the evening (after 9 p.m.) because this may result in keeping you awake well into the night. Ideally, qigong should be incorporated for at least 15 minutes of your day. However, if you are just starting, begin with once a week and slowly build up over the course of six months.

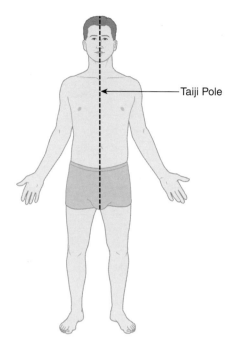

Taiji Pole

Figure 2.1 Taiji Pole.

energetic center of the body, called the *Taiji Pole*, straightened. The Taiji Pole is a column of energy extending from the top of the head at the crown down to the perineum and links all the energetic meridians and centers along the midline of the body (see figure 2.1). Each end of the Taiji Pole is an energetic portal that connects upward to Heaven and downward to Earth. Keeping the Taiji Pole straightened facilitates free-flowing qi through its core and a flowing current between the head and feet.

The second important benefit of free-flowing qi is the effect of release—in order to hold great structure, we must relax the muscles and allow the bones to hold themselves in place using minimal effort. Relaxing the muscles entails an active command from the mind to release tension, and releasing muscular tension also implies letting go of emotional and mental tension. When the entire body is relaxed, our true nature is allowed the freedom of expression.

For example, a common place to hold onto tension is the shoulders. One of the rules of posture requires the practitioner to drop the shoulders—that means don't bring them up by the ears. Let's say you've come home from a stressful day at work. It's likely that your shoulders have been creeping up toward your ears or cramping your neck. To relax the shoulders, the mental and emotional tension that put them there in the first place would also have to be released. We would have to leave our job behind and be completely whole and alone in our body. When we are on guard, we tend to hold the muscular pattern that goes with that attitude. Once we can release and fall naturally into proper alignment, the healing has already begun!

Examples of Correct Posture

Let's define proper posture beginning from the floor up. Paying close attention to these rules will ensure a safe qigong practice, lower the likelihood of injuries, and support qi flow. This is the basic posture from which most of the qigong exercises in this book will begin. For simplicity, it will be referred to as the beginning posture.

Feet

Establishing a root or connection to the Earth is important in qigong. As we perform our qigong routine, we want to visualize the body sinking into the ground and the soles of the feet opening or grabbing the Earth to facilitate an energetic exchange between the body and the ground.

A good connection to the ground is established by placing the feet shoulder width apart. This means that the centers of the feet are under the shoulder joints. Be careful to not step out too far or too narrow. Shoulder width is perfect for qi flow and is the safest distance to avoid knee injuries. Make sure your feet are parallel with each other; avoid pointing the toes in or out (pigeon toes or duck feet). Check your weight so that the feet are flat on the floor, not heavy on the outside or weighted on the inside ankle. Distribute your weight evenly between heels and toes and from inside to outside. See figure 2.2 for an example of the proper foot position.

Once the feet are balanced, the Yong Quan, or Bubbling Well, point naturally opens. This acupuncture point, known as KD 1, is located just behind the toes in the soft part of the sole (see figure 2.3). Using your thumb, it's easy to find the hole. The energetic flow of this point is up toward the Kidneys, and through it the body is fed with healthy yin energy. When the feet are well balanced and the body is in correct alignment, this area will noticeably expand, and you will be able to feel how the muscles on the inside of the legs are activated.

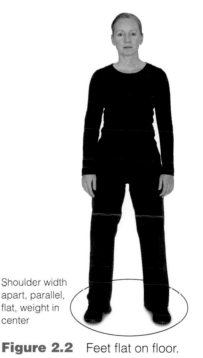

Shoulder width apart, parallel, flat, weight in center

Figure 2.2 Feet flat on floor.

By contrast (yin always has a yang), the yang meridians, which drain into the ground, are also activated, and one then has a great connection to Earth. This is called a *root* and it facilitates *grounding* (we will talk more about yin and yang and meridians in chapter 3). Grounding is important in qigong since human energy has a tendency to rise, especially when we spend so much time thinking rather than feeling. Grounding brings us back in the body where we can feel ourselves again so we can take care of our health.

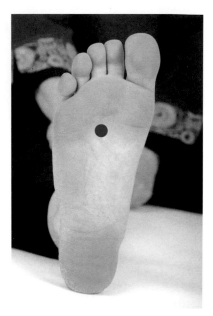

Figure 2.3 KD 1 or Bubbling Well point.

Knees

The most common injury in qigong is to the knees. Proper alignment throughout qigong practice makes a huge difference in how qi flows and reduces the likelihood of injuries. Begin by making sure to slightly bend the knees. Locked knees impede qi flow and create stress injuries on the tendons. Align the knees so that they are over the feet. Take a look at the kneecaps and make sure they are pointing straight ahead and in alignment with the toes of the feet. See figure 2.4 for an example of the proper knee position. Sagging knees into the center or twisting to the sides stresses the tendons and ligaments and greatly increases the probability of injury. The feeling is of slightly pushing the kneecaps away from each other, as in a reverse squeeze, or holding a ball between the knees. It may take a while for strength to develop, but practice will quickly change that.

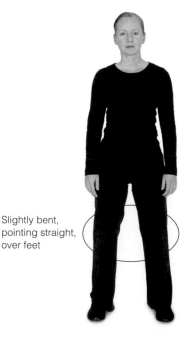

Slightly bent, pointing straight, over feet

Figure 2.4 Knees over feet.

Hips

Once the feet and knees are in the correct position, the hips tend to follow along nicely. However, make sure that the left and right sides are equal distance from the floor. If one side tends to rise more than the other, this is your first clue as to where some healing needs to begin. Next, relax the muscles. Too much attention on holding the posture will sometimes create tension. Find the place that feels comfortable and then relax. Bring your attention to the sacrum and tuck the tailbone under slightly so that the sacrum is somewhat more vertical, softening the curve on the lower lumbar region. This naturally brings in the lower belly and straightens the lower spine. Finally, softly tighten the anal sphincter. This rounds the pelvic floor and helps to avoid qi loss from the lower dantian and avoids hemorrhoids in people with sinking qi (figure 2.5). (There are three dantian—upper, middle, and lower—which are energetic centers of the body that store and distribute qi. These will be discussed in more detail in chapter 3).

Shoulders

The next area of attention is the upper torso. Begin by bringing your awareness to the center of your chest. Is it sunken toward the spine? Lift the front of the chest so that you're not slouching, naturally stretching the spine erect and upward. Check the back between the scapulas and pull the shoulders slightly forward so you can feel the band stretch around the back. Let the shoulders naturally descend, releasing any tension in the trapezius muscles. Finally, check your alignment by sensing the armpits, allowing the arms to create a hollow between the upper ribs and the arms (figure 2.6).

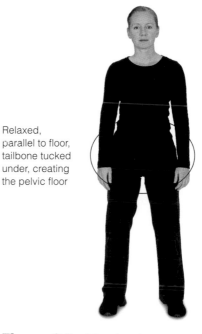

Relaxed, parallel to floor, tailbone tucked under, creating the pelvic floor

Figure 2.5 Hips level.

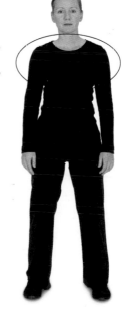

Tucked-in chest, rounded back, shoulders down, hollowed armpit

Figure 2.6 Shoulders relaxed.

Arms

With the shoulders naturally released and relaxed, the arms will also relax into a smooth posture, free from sharp bends. Let them hang without tension by the sides of the body. The elbows naturally point toward the ground or toward the back, not to the left or right (figure 2.7). Let the hand find a comfortable extended position where the wrist is not tense. There will be a natural sloping curve from the shoulder to the tips of the fingers.

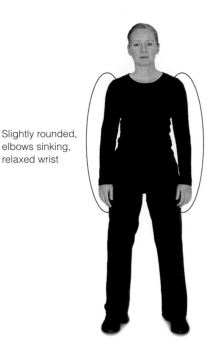

Slightly rounded, elbows sinking, relaxed wrist

Figure 2.7 Curve the elbows.

Head

Visualize the crown of the head (Bai Hui point) reaching up to Heaven. This will extend the neck, stretching the cervical vertebrae. Tuck in the chin and tilt the head slightly down, which naturally lifts the occiput (back of the head) higher. By the time the body is in complete alignment and the chin is tucked in, you should feel a continuous, smooth, stretching, lifting feeling from the sacrum to the top of the head (figure 2.8). It is commonly described as being suspended from Heaven by a thread. At this point, bring your awareness inward, avoiding reaction and processing of environmental stimuli. Touch your tongue to the roof of the mouth behind the teeth, thus connecting the Governing Vessel to the Conception Vessel (see Governing and Conception Vessels on page 18 for more information).

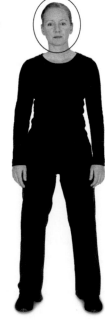

Tucked-in chin, awareness inward, tongue touched to upper palate

Figure 2.8 Lift the back and tuck the chin.

Governing and Conception Vessels

The Governing and Conception Vessels are two major energetic channels that run along the midline of the body, dividing it into right and left sides. The Governing Vessel naturally distributes qi in an ascending manner up the back of the body along the spine from the tip of the tailbone to the inside of the mouth. The Conception Vessel naturally distributes qi in an ascending manner up the front of the body from the area of the perineum to the bottom jaw.

These two important vessels have several functions, including feeding yin and yang qi into all the other meridians. If the Governing and Conception Vessels are strong and full, then they provide a good foundation on which to address more subtle merdians. For this reason, great emphasis is placed on ensuring proper alignment of the spine, head, and hips while practicing qigong.

Once the body is in correct alignment, as shown in figure 2.9, qi flow is almost immediately activated. The cells and skin of the body come alive, and it feels as if the entire body is buzzing with energy. Holding this posture for a few minutes can be a qigong practice itself in that there is an active flow of energy up the feet and the inside of the legs and down the outside of the legs. If one activates the body above the hips by bringing awareness to the correct alignment in the torso, the posture also includes qi flow through the Governing and Conception Vessels and three dantian. Once the torso is activated, qi will fill the body and flow into the arms. If the neck is slightly stretched and reaching for Heaven, then the entire body will feel alive. Take some time to discover this posture; find places where the body feels empty and adjust your posture to activate it. If a particular area is difficult to access, just take your time with it— it's possible there is an old injury (or recent one!). Allow your body to slowly unfold and relax into each section.

The same rules of alignment apply even when moving. There will be times when the arms or legs may appear to be completely straightened; however, the elbows or knees are never locked in place. As you move through a qigong routine, try to maintain the feeling of expansion and release that you discovered in the beginning posture. Keeping a slow pace will enable you to constantly check and make adjustments as necessary.

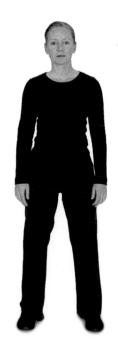

Figure 2.9 Beginning posture.

Qigong is a lot about letting go. As you work through the basics of posture, imagine your muscles relaxing and releasing tension. Allow your body to rest comfortably in the alignment as explained previously. The less tension created by your muscles, the more qi is able to flow through the meridians. The more open your joints are and the more relaxed your breathing is while holding this posture, the more you will feel qi flowing at a deeper level. In fact, you may feel heat or tingling right away. It's perfectly normal and a confirmation that your qi is moving!

Even if you practice for your entire lifetime, it's to be expected that you'll always be checking your alignment. In fact, you'll notice that as you become stronger in one area, your overall alignment will shift. Then, as you gain confidence in holding a particular posture, the challenge will be to let the muscles relax and open. The key to finding good posture in qigong is to allow these changes to take place and not get frustrated if something is challenging. The body is learning each time you practice, and even minute shifts can often translate into big results. Be patient and allow the journey to unfold.

As you gain confidence in your posture, remember to let go on all levels: body, breath, and mind. Let go of the pressure to do it right the first time; let go of the need to feel immediate results; let go of the internal critic who points out all the obstacles that are in the way of correct alignment; let go of wondering what others are thinking about you; and let go of stress. Let go, let go, let go… It's quite a wonderful feeling!

Chapter 3

Breath

We now begin our exploration into what is meant by *breath*. We will also learn about the major energetic centers in the body and the meridians that distribute qi. The key to an exhilarating qigong practice lies in understanding what qi is and how to work with it. Once we understand how qi affects the body, it will be easier to grasp the purpose of the qigong presented in this book.

This level of defining qigong, *breath*, relates to the second realm of the Three Treasures of our being, or more specifically, qi. Among the many translations or connotations of the Chinese word *qi*, one of the most popular is "breath." This definition implies the movement of air in and out of the lungs. It is one of the most basic and perhaps concrete definitions, but that does not take away from its importance. The expanding and contracting action of the lungs pumps both oxygen and qi but also stimulates and supports the heart. In fact, the heart and lungs are sometimes seen as emulating the interaction of yin and yang because their constant contraction and expansion support each others' rhythm.

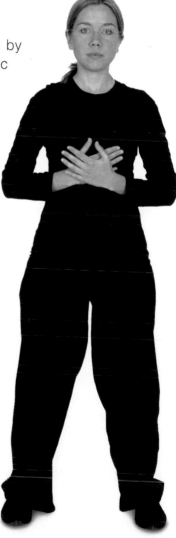

Qi as Breath

For a qigong routine to be effective, coordinating the flow of breath with the body action is essential. In general, inhalations and exhalations are matched perfectly to the length and timing of an arm or leg movement. For example, if the qigong movement involves making a circle, the inhalation would be one half of the circle and the exhalation would be the other half. This is referred to as matching the breath to the movement. For other movements or qigong exercises, the breath rate may increase or decrease. There may be instances in which several repetitions of arm or leg movements will be performed during a single drawn-out breath. But there will always be a repetitive rhythm that can be matched to a breathing pattern, making it easy to identify when to inhale and exhale.

What is the best way to breathe while practicing qigong?

Natural breathing, the way the chest and belly normally fill when we breathe in a relaxed state, is the best way to practice qigong. To practice natural breathing, simply inhale and exhale through the nose. If necessary, inhale through the nose and exhale through the mouth. It's OK to take small breaths between movements if necessary.

As we go forward into each qigong move, you will be instructed when to inhale and exhale. In the beginning, you may find it difficult to maintain the rhythm of breath matched to the movement, and it may be necessary to take a small breath in the middle of a particular move. It's OK to do that, but try to build up to following the prescribed breathing pattern throughout all the repetitions because it is then that the maximum benefit is obtained. Remember that qigong has been practiced for thousands of years, and the particular breathing pattern for each exercise often has multiple layers of meaning and purpose.

Naturally, the mechanics of breathing are important, but another way to benefit from inhalations and exhalations is to visualize them as bringing in healthy qi and releasing toxic qi. We can visualize qi entering or exiting the body in the form of colors, substance, or intention (chapter 4 will go into more detail on how to do so). When practicing qigong for health, we usually use an inhalation to *tonify*, or add healthy qi to the body. Inhalations are also generally performed when doing a motion that is either lifting or expanding so the breath is used to support the feeling of opening, stretching, and filling. On the other hand, exhalations are generally used to *purge*, or remove pathogens from the body. Exhalations are often associated with sinking or contracting motions to support the feelings and intention of releasing, draining, or emptying.

Remembering the following simple associations for breathing can make a big difference in the effectiveness of your routine:

▶ Inhale and exhale through the nose, not the mouth. If necessary, inhale through the nose and exhale through the mouth.

► Keep the timing of the breath smooth and consistent.

► Match the inhalation and exhalation to the exercise.

► Inhale to add, or tonify, and associate with expanding or lifting movements.

► Exhale to remove, or purge, and associate with contracting or sinking movements.

Qi is more than just the mechanics of breathing, however; it is also the subtle energy that we discussed in chapter 1. Now that you know how to hold the body in correct alignment and the basics of inhaling and exhaling, it's time to learn what the breath is doing on an energetic level. The following is a brief introduction to some core concepts that will put your qigong routine into context.

Qi as Energy

Qi is the energy of all things included in the Three Treasures; it is the life force of all humans, the mystical connection to the entire cosmos. The literal translation of the word *qi* from Chinese is "breath," but the meaning in Chinese implies a three-dimensional concept that includes the ability to transport a charge from one place to another; therefore, it also implies movement. The capacity of qi to transport charges through the body means that what is generated in one area can be relocated to another. Qi carries light, thought, emotion, sound, and intention to all parts of the body, affecting how each part of our being acts or reacts. Understanding the pathways through which qi moves and the energetic centers where it is generated will give great insight into the structure of your qigong routine.

When we practice qigong, we are affecting our bodies on all these levels at the same time, creating the possibility for great health and healing. When qi flows, we are releasing, relaxing, and rejuvenating each cell and allowing the opportunity for more of the strength of who we are to shine through. It is for this reason that qigong results in incredible accomplishments in the field of health care.

Qi is the life force carried in the Blood. It travels in and over the veins like mist over a river on a humid morning. It is also carried throughout the body in other types of rivers called *meridians*. These meridians are energetic pathways that nourish each part of the body with qi. For over 3,000 years, it has been known that qi travels in these meridians in a fixed pattern and direction. Qigong relies on the distribution of qi through the meridians to accomplish its great healing. Qigong practitioners commonly describe qi movement as tingling, buzzing, wind, cold, hot, or vibration. With time and practice, one can become very sensitive to qi traveling throughout the body.

Is qi in the body purely a Chinese concept?

No, the concept of qi exists in many cultures around the world. It is known as prana, ka, ki, energy, and more, and it is recognized by shamans, medicine healers, spiritual leaders, tribes, and ancient cultures from all continents.

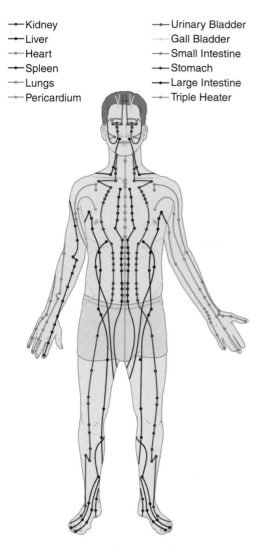

Kidney
Liver
Heart
Spleen
Lungs
Pericardium

Urinary Bladder
Gall Bladder
Small Intestine
Stomach
Large Intestine
Triple Heater

Figure 3.1   Twelve qi meridians.

The source of each meridian is a major organ that also gives the meridian its name (see figure 3.1). The meridians are divided into yin and yang. The yin organs and corresponding meridians are the Heart, Spleen, Lungs, Kidneys, Liver, and Pericardium. Each yin organ has a paired yang organ, and the corresponding meridians are the Small Intestine, Stomach, Large Intestine, Urinary Bladder, Gall Bladder, and Triple Heater.

Going back to the example of the flowing river, if we visualize the organs as a natural spring continuously pouring out water, then the metaphorical stream where the water flows in would be the meridian of that organ. Therefore, there are 12 meridians, which have the same name as their source organ. The meridians flow up and down the arms, legs, or torso. Together, the organs and meridians distribute and balance yin and yang energy throughout the body. This qi network plays an important role in how qigong moves are developed and why they are practiced in a certain manner.

All the meridians are nourished by the *Taiji Pole*. The Taiji Pole is an energetic link between Heaven and Earth that runs through the core of the body. It is a powerful energy source and can be visualized as a thick beam of light connecting the top of the head and the center of the perineum.

The Taiji Pole nourishes the three major energetic centers of the body, called *dantian*. The dantian serve as main processing points for particular types of energy. The lower dantian is located in the center of the pelvic region and is related to kinesthetic, or physical, energy. It is commonly mentioned in qigong because it is considered the beginning place for storing and cultivating qi. The middle dantian is in the center of the chest and is related to emotional, or feeling, energy. And the upper dantian is in the center of the head and is related to mental, or thinking, energy.

Together, all the qi emitted by these energetic centers and pathways creates an energetic aura called *wei qi* (*wei* means "external"). The wei qi fields are subtle energetic bubbles that extend beyond the skin, wrapping the body in a protective shield. Wei qi is further classified into three layers according to its thickness and proximity to the body. Each wei qi field also relates to a dantian. The first wei qi

Yang Versus Yin Qi

If qi is the energy that permeates the universe and is part of everything, then the names *yin* and *yang* are adjectives that describe the qualities of qi. Differentiating between the two is merely a matter of putting one in contrast to the other. It's a practice in relativity, such as in the way we know something is cold is by comparing it with something that is hot, or we know something is heavy because we've already experienced something that is light. Yang is merely describing something that is harder, heavier, or external compared with something that is softer, lighter, and internal (yin).

In qigong practice, yang energy would include fast movements, stomping, clapping, or shouting, whereas yin energy would include slow movements, meditation, and quietness. To truly understand the difference, take some time to describe objects according to the yin–yang polarity chart provided in figure 3.2. With time it will become easier to translate the knowledge into more subtle energies such as emotions and thoughts.

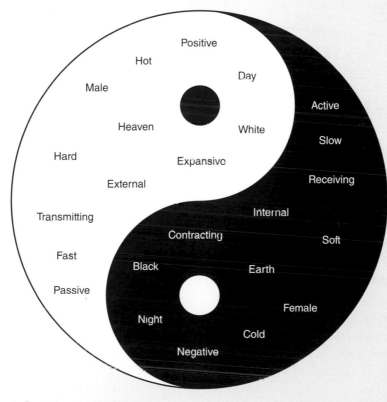

Figure 3.2 Yin–yang polarity.

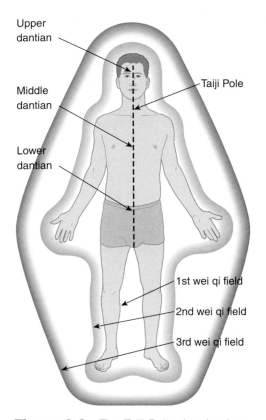

Upper dantian

Middle dantian

Lower dantian

Taiji Pole

1st wei qi field

2nd wei qi field

3rd wei qi field

Figure 3.3 The Taiji Pole, the dantian, and the wei qi fields.

field is related to the lower dantian (jing), the second wei qi field is related to the middle dantian (qi), and the third wei qi field is related to the upper dantian (shen), which will be discussed in the next chapter. It is through the wei qi fields that humans communicate with others (people, animals, and plants) nonverbally. Similar to our bodies, the wei qi fields also accumulate charges and need to be cleansed. A natural benefit of practicing qigong is the automatic cleansing and strengthening of the wei qi fields. With enough practice, one can become sensitive to shifts in the wei qi fields and thereby empowered to make any necessary adjustments.

Returning to the concept of qi, we recognize that all stimuli to the body have an energetic charge, including food, emotions, and environmental and spiritual sources. Qi charges then flow throughout all the energetic centers of the body, including the dantian, organs, meridians, Taiji Pole, and wei qi fields (figure 3.3). Throughout the day we process millions of qi stimuli. Normally, these energetic charges are moved and transformed, and we enjoy average health. However, in certain instances the energetic charge is stored in the organs or tissues and begins to draw in additional energy to support its particular energetic qualities. If that matrix is continuously fed or supported over time with similar energy, it can then grow and develop into disease. Let's look at an example to further put this information in context.

A man worked diligently at a place of employment for years, giving up many family moments for it and enduring office politics, long hours, and personal conflicts, all with the vision of one day receiving a promotion. Then, one day he was late and forgot to call the boss. That day, he was fired. What was his reaction? A lot of anger. It's a normal response to a situation that was out of his control. That's the energetic charge. It would also be normal for the anger to pass after a short time. However, let's say that for some reason it didn't, and this man plotted ways in which he could take revenge on the company and perhaps even the boss. That's the energy that feeds the initial charge and begins to create a cycle. This man's anger now remains unresolved and somewhat present but not specifically directed at the trigger factor (boss/company). Now, he's driving around and is angry with other drivers, and he has a short temper at home and takes it out on the kids. Furthermore, he decides that alcohol may be the way to deal with the stress of all these problems, so he begins to spend time at the local bar.

The man may not realize what is happening and maybe doesn't even see the link between all these actions; however, little by little a problem is developing. Each incident of anger, irritation, and drinking is feeding the original anger, and the reinforcement only exacerbates the problem. It slowly creates a cycle that can lead to health problems related to the Liver. The emotion of anger is related to the Liver, and when the Liver is out of balance, a person can display anger and irritation.

How can this man turn this energy around? Because he is stressed, his doctor recommends he start a qigong class. At first, it's hard to relax and drop into the movements, especially the breath, but once he begins to move the energy around and consciously invoke relaxing and releasing, he can feel little pieces of anger fall away. After a month, he is no longer angry at traffic, his home relationships have improved, and he's facing the trigger factor (losing his job) with a new perspective. Without the charges holding that anger, he can begin to open up and explore new possibilities. Internally, the cluster of energetic charge has been broken up and no longer binds to his tissues; the qi is released and flow is occurring once again.

To summarize, the way we think and feel can change the way we breathe and how qi flows through the body, and over time it can have an effect on our health. The good news is that we can control these effects by becoming conscious of our breathing patterns and the places where we hold onto qi. Ultimately, the goal is to identify the stimulus as it happens and to take preventive measures instead of waiting until the effects are longer term. The next step is to integrate body and breath into mind. It is in the realm of mind or spirit that qigong begins to develop into more than just an exercise.

Chapter 4

Intention

The most abstract component of qigong practice relates to the mind, or intention. The mind is a powerful part of our being, and with it we are capable of accomplishing incredible tasks. Some of these tasks we are aware of, such as thinking and processing data, and others remain to be discovered, such as controlling and directing qi. Because qigong depends a great deal on mental visualizations, learning how to guide our thoughts and intentions is a key element of a successful practice.

This level of defining qigong, *intention*, relates to the third level of the Three Treasures of our being, or more specifically, shen. The mind's intention is closely associated with, and sometimes interpreted as, shen. Although shen and intention are not exactly the same, they are both the most abstract and ethereal parts of our being. We will explore the relationship between the two in the next few paragraphs.

In addition to posture and breath, a successful qigong practice depends on integrating the mind. One way of doing that is through the use of intention. Simply stated, intention is the object of our visualization; in other words, it's what we're thinking about when doing qigong. One of the fundamental tenets of qigong is that intention guides the qi. What this means and how to practice it plays a crucial part in the effectiveness of qigong practice. Each qigong practice can take on a completely different feeling or meaning simply by changing the intention. In terms of qigong for health, the object of our mind's visualization while we practice determines the effect the movement of qi will have on our health. Changing the direction means that the mind is changing the current pattern and flow of qi, and by changing the flow of qi, we can create change at the level of tissues, muscles, and bones. The mind guides the qi, and the qi guides the jing.

Let's take a quick look at shen. Shen is commonly thought of as the spiritual aspect of the person and is associated with the upper dantian and mental capacities. This concept was first introduced in chapter 1 when we discussed the Three Treasures. People practicing qigong for spiritual purposes would focus much attention on the development of shen as well as qi and jing. For people practicing qigong for purposes other than a spiritual path, the mental aspect is considered *intention*.

Another way to distinguish between shen and intention is as follows: Shen exists as an energy that is inherent in every human being and is independent of a particular faith. Faith could be considered an intention that is given to the shen for direction. In qigong for health, which is the purpose of this book, our intention is to promote healing, and we accomplish that by focusing on the areas of our body that need to be brought into balance. Our shen is guided by the intention of health or healing we desire. Once we have established our healing intention, the qi begins to respond, and as the qi responds, so does the jing. Eventually, the body is healed according to the intention we specified. So again, intention guides the qi, which guides the jing.

Saying that the mind can alter the flow of qi to promote health implies that our mind can also be the catalyst for disease when it is caught in a destructive pattern or disassociated from the rest of the body. Deteriorating health due to chronic stress is just one example of this. The best way

Are mind, intention, and shen the same thing?

Simply stated, no. They are three different concepts that are often used interchangeably to describe a process that happens mostly in the head. Your mind can be considered the thinking part of yourself, intention can be considered the object or purpose of your thoughts, and shen is literally translated as "spirit" and is the most subtle of the three energies. It is important to distinguish among them because shen is the most subtle part of our energetic anatomy, yet it has a big impact on our overall health. In order to heal or maintain great health, we must give equal importance to this part of ourselves. In order to effect change on the level of shen, we must work with the mind. Identifying thought patterns that are healthy is a way of establishing good intention, and since intention guides qi and qi guides jing, it is the most effective way of ensuring radiant health.

to keep the mind away from unhealthy patterns is to keep it relaxed and rooted in the body, free from countless distractions. A grounded mind is fundamental to maintaining great health mentally, emotionally, and physically. This requires skill and practice, but it is one of the purposes of doing qigong for health.

Naturally, the next question would be, how does one obtain a peaceful mind? In order to accomplish this it's important to understand what pulls us out of this connectedness and center. Once we know what has disconnected us, it's easy to determine how to change it. Fortunately, qigong counts on some effective tools to help us navigate the complexities of both body and mind. The next section will introduce the Five Elements cycle, a key to understanding the relationships among body, breath, and mind.

Five Elements Cycle

Now that we understand the relationship of mind and intention, we are ready to identify a purpose for our practice and to create an environment that supports it. A typical class of qigong for health often asks students to visualize vivid scenarios or movement of qi around and through the body. Colors, emotions, organs, sensations, sound, and more are all carefully put together so as to invoke the senses. The purpose of these visualizations is to trigger the flow of qi through a particular organ, meridian, or energetic center and facilitate the desired result. The practitioner's ability to integrate a vivid visualization with the corresponding breath and movement can create profound qi experiences and is ultimately the key to making any qigong routine significantly effective.

But how do we identify which intention to use? What does it do? And where do we start? To begin to answer that question, we must first understand the relationship of each energetic center with colors, sounds, emotions, and more. Understanding this relationship enables a deeper assimilation of the reason qigong is orchestrated in particular patterns or structures. The Five Elements cycle is an amazing resource that answers many of these questions.

Working with the Five Elements cycle is a profound experience. I often think of the interaction of all the energies within the Three Treasures as a three-dimensional map of the universe. To make the journey throughout the microcosm of humanity or macrocosm of the universe, one would need a compass. That compass, or the legend of the map, is the Five Elements cycle (see figure 4.1). Within the apparent simplicity of five elements—Water, Wood, Fire, Earth, and Metal—lies a vast wealth of information. Knowing how to apply each element to your qigong practice will reveal profound insight into your health and well-being.

The Five Elements embody several meanings that can be applied according to the purpose of one's practice. At face value, each element is a direct translation of its name. For example, let's take a look at Fire. Fire is exactly that—hot burning flame, traditionally kindled by wood, upward-expanding heat. But the name of the element is also a representation of the many qualities it embodies. For example,

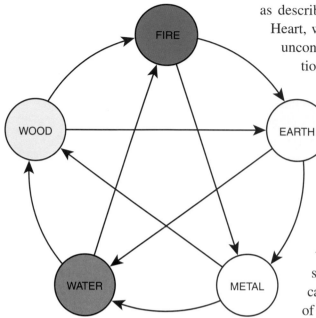

as described in table 4.1, Fire represents the Heart, which houses the spirit, the virtue of unconditional love, and the acquired emotion of overexcitement. It also represents the zenith of summer, the color red, and the south direction. This is valuable information because it means that it is possible to alter the condition of each element by working with any one of the qualities it represents.

On the other hand, if you take a look again at figure 4.1, the circle and the star indicate the energetic relationship between each element. They indicate where there is a natural ebb and flow of qi throughout the Five Elements and their corresponding meridians. The goal of TCM is to keep the qi flowing naturally among them by understanding where any blockages may be and resolving them.

Figure 4.1 The Five Elements cycle.

The arrows that form a circle symbolize the creation cycle, which states that each element nourishes the element following it. If we return to the metaphor of the river in chapter 3, where the source of the river is an organ, let's say the organ overflows and fills the river, and the river then flows downstream and eventually into the next organ. Therefore, if Fire overflows, it will nourish or create Earth. If

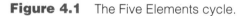

TABLE 4.1

Qualities of the Five Elements

	Fire	Earth	Metal	Water	Wood
Yin organ	Heart	Spleen	Lungs	Kidneys	Liver
Yang organ	Small Intestine	Stomach	Large Intestine	Urinary Bladder	Gall Bladder
Color	Red	Yellow/brown	White	Blue/purple or black	Blue/green
Virtue	Unconditional love	Trust	Integrity	Wisdom	Benevolence
Emotion	Overexcitement	Worry	Grief	Fear	Anger
Season	Summer	Center	Autumn	Winter	Spring

Earth overflows, it creates Metal. If the qi is flowing freely among the elements, then strengthening one element will provide a trickle-down effect of strengthening those that follow. By contrast, if there is a blockage in any organ, then it will restrict the flow of qi to the organs that follow it.

The elements also have yin and yang energies, and one way of seeing that clearly is through the emotions. On the yin side, each element represents a positive attribute, or virtue of existence; on the yang side are the negative reactions (acquired emotions) related to the experience of living. The balance of yin and yang energy in the body's energetic centers is important because spending too much time out of balance can create chronic diseases. It's normal to experience shifts from yang to yin and vice versa in accordance with specific cycles or experiences; it's when the shift remains predominantly on one side or the other that defines a condition. (Note that a total balance between all elements simultaneously is unachievable, so when we speak of balance and harmony of the elements, what we mean is functioning within a normal ebb and flow.)

Let's look at an example of the creation cycle in terms of emotions and the interplay of yin and yang. In the element of Wood, the yin qi is the virtue of benevolence, and the yang qi is the emotion of anger or irritation. The Five Elements theory says that when this element is in balance, we are kind and generous and are not quick to anger. If the Wood element is out of balance on the yin side, then we are too generous and lack healthy emotional boundaries. If the Wood element is out of balance on the yang side, then we become irritable and prone to fits of anger, and we lack generosity. To restore harmony between yin and yang by using the elements, we could strengthen (tonify) the Wood element directly, or we could strengthen it indirectly by strengthening the Water element, which would overflow and nourish Wood. Note that the Daoist Five qigong set, which we will learn in chapter 6, goes through each of the elements and shows a specific qigong move for promoting change in the corresponding organ.

The following sections provide a closer look at each element individually.

Metal

Metal corresponds to the Lungs (yin organ) and Large Intestine (yang organ). When in a balanced state it is expressed as the virtue of Integrity and the ability to let go of attachments. The emotions of grief or sorrow are expressions of the Metal element as well as conditions of the lungs which obstruct breathing, such as asthma and bronchitis. The Metal element is represented by the color white for purity and activated in the "sh" sound. In the body it is reflected in the skin, body hair, nose, and the action of crying. It relates to the season of autumn and is supported by the West direction, foods that are pungent, and metal objects. The qualities of metal in people are sharp, focused, determined, and persistent. They also tend to be future oriented, organized, and minimalistic yet interested in wealth and simple luxuries. The energy of Metal is "contracting."

Water

Water corresponds to the Kidneys (yin organ) and the Urinary Bladder (yang organ). When in a balanced state it is expressed as the virtue of Wisdom and the ability to face life's many situations with confidence and courage. The emotion of fear, including that of not having, being, or doing enough, drains the Kidneys and consumes the Water reserves which are accumulated during the season of winter. Its associated color is black, which represents the feeling of deep introspection, listening, quiet, stillness, conserving, dormancy, and the essence of Yin. The Water element is activated with the "chree" sound and is expressed by groaning. In the body it is reflected in the quality of the fluids, the strength of the bones, and the acuteness of hearing. It is associated with the North direction, foods that are salty, and all bodies of water. People who display Water element personalities tend to be introverted with a strong desire for contemplating truth and wisdom; they are strong willed and are interested in deep, contemplative conversation or philosophy. The energy of Water is "conserving."

Wood

Wood corresponds to the Liver (yin organ) and Gall Bladder (yang organ). When in a balanced state, it is expressed as the virtue of Kindness and Benevolence and the inspiration viewing life with the creative passion of "anything is possible." When out of balance, the Wood element becomes rigid and inflexible, highly defensive, lashing out with anger and irritation. The Wood element flourishes in the spring in shades of blue and green when life begins to emerge from the quiet slumber of winter. The Wood element is activated with the "shu" sound (pronounced "shoo") and is expressed by shouting. In the body it is reflected in the quality and strength of the tendons and the eyes. It is associated with the East direction and foods that are sour. The energy of Wood is "creative."

Fire

Fire corresponds to the Heart (yin organ) and Small Intestine (yang organ). In some systems it also includes the Pericardium (yin) and Triple Heater (yang) meridians. When in a balanced state, Fire is confident to express itself as the virtue of Unconditional Love and the ability to offer abundance and joy. When out of balance, the Fire element becomes nervous, agitated, or over excited, consuming itself and jumping around like a blazing fire. The Fire element represents our spiritual connection, and the Heart is considered its home. So it seeks to maintain the Heart open and flowing with pure loving energy, preserving our connection to the Divine. The Fire element is the zenith of summer, during which the heat exposes life to maximum yang energy and represents the culmination of growth. The Fire element is activated with the "ha" sound and is expressed through laughter. In the body it is reflected in the quality of the Blood, perspiration, and the complexion of the face. It is associated with the Southern direction and foods that are bitter. The energy of Fire is "expanding."

Earth

Earth corresponds to the Spleen (yin organ) and Stomach (yang organ) meridians. When in a balanced state it is expressed as the virtue of Trust and Faith. The emotion of worry congeals and taxes the Spleen and can be the root of conditions such as Diabetes. The Earth element is related to the sweet taste and is represented by a mustard yellow color. It is activated by the "whoo" sound and the action of singing. In the body it is reflected in the quality of the muscles and the mouth. In terms of seasons, there are two theories: one, that it is late summer, the last burning part of summer before transitioning to autumn; the other, that it is the grounding period between each season, a time of transition from one to the other. Earth is the center of all directions. The qualities of Earth in persons are grounding, nourishing, and nurturing. They tend to be accepting of others and enjoy the pleasures of emotions, many times identifying themselves through the experience of these emotions. They can be very forgiving and open. Earth people love our planet and enjoy gardening, nature, and all that life has to offer. The energy of Earth is "transforming."

Keeping Your Practice Simple

Once you understand the principles behind the Five Elements cycle and become acquainted with the symbolic relationship of each element, then you can begin to pinpoint which area is most suitable for the intention of your practice. Remember to put the Five Elements into perspective with the Three Treasures (jing or body, qi or energy, and shen or spirit) to get a better picture of the specific energy to work with during your qigong practice. When doing so, there are a few considerations to keep in mind. The first recommendation is to *simplify the object of your focus*; the more singular our focus is at any time, the more resources we have available to support the focus. If we are trying to juggle multiple objects at one time, our energy or resources are divided into that many objects. In terms of qi, a juggling act can be exhausting, and it doesn't allow a clear message to be communicated. A practical example that demonstrates the beauty of practicing qigong is the modern lifestyle. The average person today processes and receives thousands of times more input than our ancestors did. We are in a constant state of input from work, family, traffic, exercise, recreation, TV, cell phones, reading, and texting, and the effects are devastating. We are stressed, tired, and unhealthy, and we don't know how to stop.

The very method of practicing qigong, simplifying the mind, tuning out the noise, and focusing on a single thing, taps into the beginning of the healing process. However, this is much easier said than done. Take the example of stress, an abstract and intangible thing. It could be said that to eliminate stress, all we have to do is not think about it. However, ask someone who's stressed if she can simply relax. It's difficult. By the same token, the mental aspect of qigong, which many people might assume would be the easiest, is actually the most difficult. In other words, your mind may be the biggest obstacle to overcome. But with patience and practice, it is entirely possible.

In working with the Five Elements, singular focus means selecting only one aspect to work on at a time. That is, if you will be working through all Five Elements in your qigong practice, then select only one of the rows in table 4.1. As you move through each element, the visualization of that element is simplified into virtue, emotion, color, or sound. By keeping it simple, the mind does not struggle to hold on to various visualizations, and therefore your intention is stronger and more able to effect change at the level you're working on. For example, if you decide to work on the Heart, it's easier to work on only color at the beginning than to try to focus on a combination of direction, sound, meridians, emotions, and so on all at the same time.

Another consideration to keep in mind is *consistency*. Consistency means that although we may be changing from one movement to another, we are still following through with the same intention. In general, this applies to being consistent while working within a particular qigong set. For example, if we are practicing the Daoist Five Yin for tonification, then we would hold the intention of tonification throughout the entire set and not jump to purging or regulating. Our visualization would be consistent throughout all the elements. If we want to change the visualization to purging, then it's best to do that at a separate practice time. Simply put, consistency supports the guideline of simplicity: Stay focused and avoid jumping around from one thing to another.

As you begin working with intention and visualization during your practice, the most common challenge at the beginning is the wandering mind. Perhaps the first few times we approach qigong, our mind may be consumed with trying to remember all the details covered in this book, but once we begin to feel confident in how we're moving and breathing, the next challenge is to keep the mind focused and connected to the intention. Depending on our stress level and our experience with turning off the noise, it will be easier or harder to maintain a consistent level of focus throughout the routine. The same advice from previous chapters applies here—be patient and forgiving to yourself; don't create additional psychological obstacles to overcome such as frustration or self-criticism. Nobody started the journey of qigong as an expert, not even the masters high on mountaintops. Everybody starts in the same place; the difference is the willingness to stick with it despite the many challenges that arise. Qigong is a journey of self-discovery where with each day and with each revelation we are given a beautiful gift—that of understanding more about ourselves, how we view the world, and why we view it that way. We are given the opportunity to release behaviors and interpretations that limit us and instead are empowered with freedom to be the shining person we are deep inside, a spiritual being blessed with compassion, integrity, wisdom, benevolence, and love.

Now that we know how to apply the mind during qigong practice, we can move on to integrating the three components of qigong into a healing flow. First, let's review the information we've covered so far:

- ► We've learned that in order to begin practice, we must align the body to maximize the flow of qi (chapter 2, Posture).
- ► We've learned how to breathe and where the energetic centers are in the body and the pathways through which they move (chapter 3, Breath).
- ► We've learned that an abstract third layer exists to our practice, which is the intention or visualization (chapter 4, Intention).

The best way to integrate the three components of qigong (posture, breath, and intention) is to begin with posture. Don't worry about perfecting each and every posture or movement before moving on; just spend enough time working on the body so that it can comfortably support the next step. Once you have developed confidence in how you hold your body while in static or dynamic qigong, then it's time to move on to the breath. Notice your natural breathing rhythm and try to extend it to match your movements. Finally, add the intention or visualization to your qigong. With the Three Treasures moving in harmony, now you're doing qigong!

Chapter 5

Structuring a Qigong Routine

Qigong has evolved for more than 3,000 years, leading to a wealth of qigong forms. Today, there are thousands of qigong movements. Two broad categories of these movements are single exercises, which can be practiced alone, and exercises that belong to groups of preset flows, such as the Eight Silk Brocade, the Daoist Five, or even tai chi. Regardless of which type of qigong you're doing, a few guidelines can make a big difference in the effectiveness of your practice.

The simplicity and effectiveness of qigong have greatly contributed to its success, and recently, qigong practice in the United States has seen a growing interest in single qigong exercises. As a result, some qigong movements have been isolated from their original group sets and incorporated into a highly individualized practice where the person picks the movements that she is interested in doing. The growing popularity of qigong is partially due to this flexibility. However, the cumulative benefit of the preset qigong sets is lost when the exercises are practiced in isolation. In other words, you only get part of the benefit.

What is the difference between a qigong movement, set, and routine?

A qigong movement is one single exercise or motion; for example, lifting the arms above the head. A qigong set would be multiple movements put together; for example, the Daoist Five in chapter 6. A qigong routine would be the entire qigong practice time from beginning to end.

Although qigong offers the opportunity for a tailored routine, the most effective qigong routines still follow a basic structure. This simple structure facilitates the final outcome by creating a good energetic and mental environment within which to circulate qi. Whether performing a single qigong exercise or a complete set, taking time to go through all these steps will provide significantly better results and reduce the likelihood of physical injuries or qi deviation symptoms, which are physical or emotional symptoms that are the result of practicing qigong incorrectly or overpracticing. They usually indicate qi moving against a normal pattern or stuck in certain areas.

The basic structure of a qigong routine is as follows:

- ► Opening
- ► Clearing
- ► Cultivation
- ► Centering
- ► Closing

Each part of this structure has a clear purpose, as indicated by its name. As we go through each part, its purpose will be explained and a few options will be presented for you to practice. In cultivation, you'll be able to fill in with the qigong sets in chapters 6, 7, and 8 or any other qigong not included in this book. It can be a single movement or a complete set. It's up to you! Keep in mind that with the thousands of qigong movements available to choose from, those that we cover here are just the beginning and will guide you through the basics of a qigong routine.

As we proceed, remember to begin with your attention on body alignment and the movements. After you have repeated the movements a few times and have gained confidence in performing them correctly, you can add the breath. Finally, when you're ready, integrate the visualizations and intention. You are now ready to begin moving and doing qigong!

What is the difference between tai chi and qigong?

They are similar in that they are both internally focused and work with breath, posture, and intention simultaneously. In practice, however, there are some characteristics that can begin to separate one from the other. Tai chi is a preset flow of movements in which the practitioner moves both the arms and the legs. Tai chi was developed by specific families who gave their names to the styles; for instance, Yang style came from the Yang family and Chen style came from the Chen family. The preset flows of tai chi include as many as 108 movements and for the most part can also be used for martial purposes. Qigong forms come from many sources and are generally practiced while standing or sitting in one place. Although qigong has forms that include multiple movements, in general it is isolated to single movements that can be done once or repeated multiple times.

Opening

The opening is the first moment we have to come back into our body and bring our awareness to harmonizing the Three Treasures. It creates a conscious break from our daily activities and is the transition into practicing qigong itself. It's a mental transition as much as an opportunity to put the body in proper alignment and begin regulating the breath. The opening also has the purpose of establishing a connection to Earth, or grounding. Grounding is important in that it gives our energy a place to be released. By the time your body is in alignment as described in chapter 2, you should already be running a circuit between Heaven, your body, and the Earth. The opening further reinforces that connection.

As we learned in the previous chapter, the mental aspect of qigong is equally as important as the breath and the body. Because the intention guides the qi, a calm, focused mind is essential to practicing qigong; scattered thoughts disperse qi and do not support harmony among the Three Treasures. For this same reason, the opening plays a big part in the effectiveness of any qigong routine.

Some people have stated that it's not necessary to have an opening in qigong; however, the added value of taking the time to perform an opening is substantial and makes a huge difference in the long term. Let's look at it from another point of view. A person arrives at class after work, and instead of performing the opening, he decides to just jump right into the qigong. It would take at least a few moments or repetitions for the mind, breath, and body to come into alignment. The person would perhaps be a good way into the routine before he felt an overall sense of harmony, which means that the first few repetitions were not doing their targeted purpose. Instead, these repetitions performed the function of an opening, missing the benefit they were designed to provide. Wouldn't it be better to take the time for an opening?

There are several ways to open a qigong routine. Pulling Down Heavens is the one I use the most because it's flexible and embraces several levels of the mind, breath, and body. The exercise itself is simple; its magic lies in the visualization. As an opening, Pulling Down Heavens has the focus of bringing qi down through the front, back, and middle of the body both internally and externally. The breath and arms first gather qi from the Earth and Heavens and then guide the qi in a descending motion by performing a circular motion with the arms from the top of the head through the body and down the legs. The visualization supports the feeling of being rooted in the grounding qi of Earth and bathed in the pure qi of Heaven. Blending the two above the head, one is also connected to the Divine as much as grounded in the Earth's embrace.

This Heaven–Human–Earth link is essential because it creates an energetic circuit that remains throughout the routine. Each inhalation and exhalation blurs the sensation of being separated from the environment and enhances our feeling of peace and centeredness. The downward-washing qi releases any turbid qi that may be in our presence and restores a greater connection to our internal light. Pulling Down Heavens is practiced in sets of three repetitions each.

Pulling Down Heavens

1 Start in beginning posture, palms facing the Earth. Take a few moments to settle into your body. Bring your attention to the center of the palms and begin to feel a cloud of qi develop between your palms and the Earth. Feel your hands become like suction cups with which you'll begin to pull up qi from the Earth as you inhale and begin to lift the arms.

2 Continue to inhale and lift the hands until approximately at waist height, and then slowly turn the palms over to face the Heavens. As the palms turn, the Earth qi is still in the palms, but now you're adding Heaven qi to it. Gather both Earth and Heaven qi as you inhale, bringing the hands up over the head. The arms rise at an angle of 45 degrees to your sides, not on a straight line all the way left and right. Continue lifting the arms until they are extended over the head, palms facing each other. The movement from palms facing the Earth to extended over the head corresponds to one continuous inhalation.

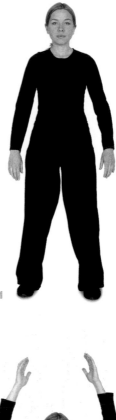

1

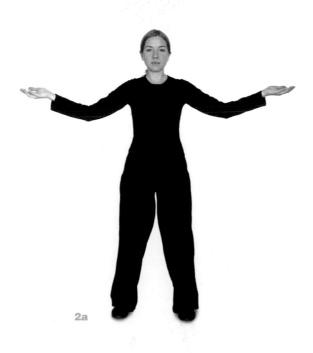

2a

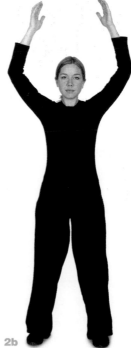

2b

3 **As you begin to exhale, let the palms turn downward, facing the body. Exhale in one continuous breath until the hands are down by the hips, completing one repetition.**

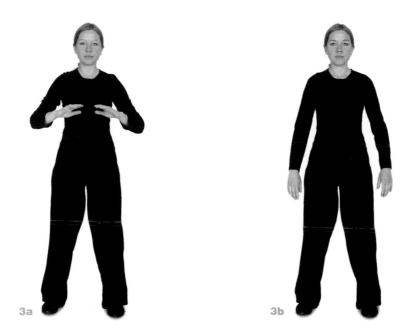

3a   3b

Pulling Down Heavens as an opening can be repeated up to three times for a total of nine repetitions. This number of repetitions is acceptable for most physical conditions. If you want to increase the number of repetitions above nine, keep in mind that this higher number is not suitable for people with low blood pressure, abundant menstruation, diarrhea, or any condition where there is excessive downward-moving qi. Note that Pulling Down Heavens can also be practiced alone as a quick pick-me-up during the day. Try doing a set of nine Pulling Down Heavens anytime you feel stressed, overloaded, or scattered. Or, teach it to your children to help them settle down before doing homework, before going to bed, or anytime they need to regroup.

Now that we have explained the movements and breathing, let's add the visualization. Each time we descend and exhale, the visualization changes from the front of the body to the center of the body to the back of the body.

Front

Visualize a shower of blended Earth and Heaven qi washing down the front of your body like a white crystal rain, clearing through the front of your face, your throat, and your chest. Allow the clean qi to penetrate into the deeper layers of the front of your body, accessing the outside of the organs as you descend. Let the clean qi wash down the front of your legs, finally draining into the Earth. See anything you want to release being absorbed by this white rain. As more and more turbidity is removed from your tissues and organs, visualize the water turning gray and feel it being pulled away from you and draining into the ground, clearing away any residue.

Center

Visualize a shower of blended Earth and Heaven qi washing down the inside of your body like a white crystal rain from the top of your head, clearing the inside of your head, the inside of your throat, and the inside of your chest. Allow the clean qi to penetrate the Taiji Pole that connects the three dantian and wash away any turbidity that is inside your body. As the qi descends, it carries away anything you want to release down the inside of the legs and finally into the Earth. See anything you want to release being absorbed by this white rain. As more and more turbidity is removed from your tissues and organs, visualize the water turning gray and feel it being pulled away from you and draining into the ground, clearing away any residue.

Back

Visualize a shower of blended Earth and Heaven qi washing down the back of your body like a white crystal rain from the top of your head, clearing the back of your head, your neck, your back, and your shoulders. Allow the clean qi to penetrate the skin, ribs, spine, and hips and wash away any turbidity that is inside or on top of your body. As the qi descends, it carries away anything you want to release down the rear of the legs and finally into the Earth. See anything you want to release being absorbed by this white rain. As more and more turbidity is removed from your tissues and organs, visualize the water turning gray and feel it being pulled away from you and draining into the ground, clearing away any residue.

Clearing

After establishing a good connection between Heaven and Earth and performing a superficial clearing of the body, our focus shifts to more specific areas such as the meridians and organs. The next few exercises will guide you through cleansing the organs, the fasciae, the meridians, and the wei qi fields. Clearing before beginning to practice qigong helps to remove any turbid qi that may be close to the surface. It is not considered a deep-focused practice but rather a general washing away of sludge. The sludge is like the dust that settles on a table when it hasn't been used in a while. During our day-to-day activities, we pick up and generate qi that doesn't necessarily serve our highest good. This qi is an accumulation of our thoughts, our emotions, the food we eat, any medication or supplements we consume, our environment, and the people or objects we come in contact with. By performing a clearing, we have the chance to get rid of the sludge and start working on a clean canvas. The following exercises can be done individually or combined for maximum effect.

Channel Dredging

Just as the name implies, this simple clearing exercise targets the meridians to clear away any turbid qi. The visualization is comparable to clearing away the bottom of a dirty riverbed where sediment and heavier objects are deposited. While performing Channel Dredging, your fingers become large scoops that rake through the meridians, clearing away any turbidity or sludge.

The exercise is divided into two parts in order to address the direction of yin and yang flow in the arms and legs, and the completion of both parts equals one repetition. Channel Dredging is usually practiced in sets of three repetitions. It is common to feel chills or electric tingling sensations throughout the arms or spine when doing this exercise. This is due to the stimulation of the meridians that run close to the surface of the skin.

PART I: Clearing the Yang Channels

1 **Start in the beginning posture. Bring your arms together so that they cross at the wrists, palms down.**

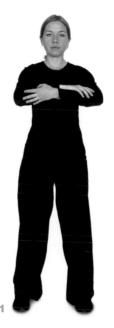

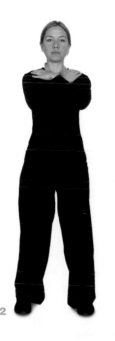

2 **Turn your hands so that they face and grasp the forearms. Turn the fingertips down so that they can rake through the meridian as the hands travel up the arms to the shoulders and stop at the base of the neck. Use your intention to grab the qi on the surface as you rise. This entire motion is accompanied by one single inhalation.**

(continued)

Channel Dredging *(continued)*

3 Keeping your hands crossed at the back of the neck, lift from the elbows so that you can rake the sides of the head. Note that each hand will be on the opposite side of the head (left hand on right side, right hand on left side). This motion allows for clearing the yang meridians that are in the head, specifically the Gall Bladder channel, which you will now access to drain the turbid qi. The hands are crossed behind the head at the occiput.

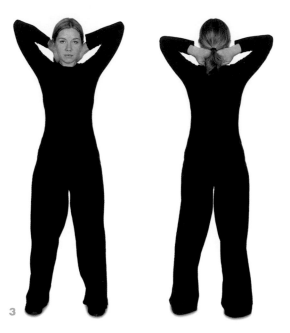

3

4 Switch to an exhalation and use your intention to guide the qi from the occiput to the shoulders. At this point you must disconnect your hands from your body and bring your palms to wrap around the rib cage, fingers pointing to the spine, and with one long sweeping motion guide the qi all the way downward to the toes and into the floor. Use the exhalation to guide the qi down the yang channels and into the Earth. Be sure to release anything that you gathered; this is qi that you want to let go of.

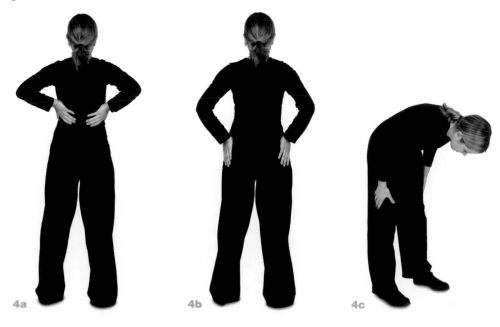

4a   4b   4c

5 One way of ending this exhalation that emphasizes the release is to make a flicking gesture with the hands after swiping the feet, similar to wiping mud off your legs and then using one strong flick of the hands to clean the mud off them. Visualize the turbid qi being sucked into the ground. Don't worry—Mother Earth will purify it for you!

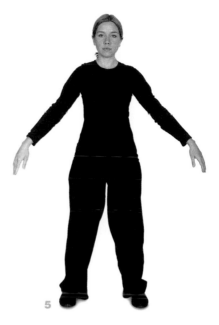

PART II: Clearing the Yin Channels

The second part of Channel Dredging is the upward sweep, which clears the yin channels. The energy of the yin meridians runs on the front and insides of the body. By clearing through both the yang and yin meridians, turbid qi is removed and qi flow is stimulated.

1 Begin with your palms facing the inside of each foot next to the arch. Do not cross the arms.

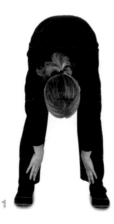

(continued)

Channel Dredging *(continued)*

2 As you inhale, use your hands to rake up through the inside of the legs. Be sure to sweep your hands up at the crease of the thighs at the hips. This ensures you are following the yin path.

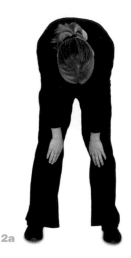

2a

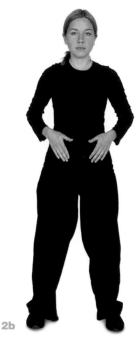

2b

3 Continue to rake up into the abdomen parallel to the midline until just under the sternum, near the center of the middle dantian.

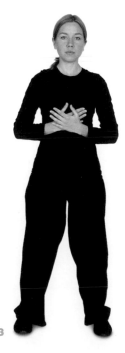

3

4 In the middle dantian area, your arms switch from a pulling action to a pushing action simultaneously as your hands begin to cross over the midline until your hands are on opposite sides in the crease of the arms.

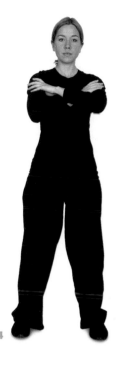

4

5 Switch to an exhalation and guide your hands down the inside of the arms all the way to the fingertips. Again, end with the flicking motion, clearing your hands of any turbid qi.

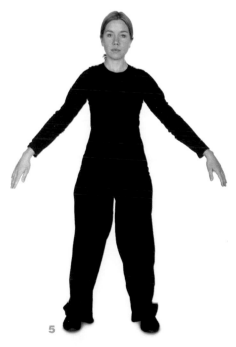

5

Counter Swing

This exercise is a great way to get the blood moving due to its quicker pace and pumping action. Qi is brought up from the Earth through the center of the legs and the torso and then released down the arms and through the palms via rhythmic swinging motions to each side.

Counter Swing is usually repeated for a total of 18 times on each side. A certain pace will build as you get used to filling and releasing. Work at a pace that feels comfortable but allows the arms to swing fairly naturally. Some common mistakes in this exercise are overextending (leaning too far forward) when releasing the qi, turning the knees too much while twisting, and holding too much tension in the muscles. Avoid holding the center position as a break between each side, yet be sure to complete the exercise as described.

1 **Start in the beginning posture. Inhale and bring the arms up to shoulder height, palms down. Remember to keep the shoulders relaxed and avoid lifting them up toward the ears. Keep the elbows pointed toward the floor and slightly bent. The overall feeling should be relaxed and loose; there should be no tension moving from the center of the chest toward the fingertips. It may take time to develop this level of relaxation. Just keep telling the muscles to relax and let go. Each time you inhale, visualize qi rising through the legs, flowing and filling the torso. When the entire torso is full of qi, it will naturally overflow into the arms. The natural response would be to allow the qi to tip the hands in the opposite direction.**

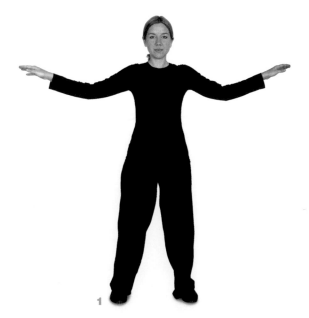

1

2 Begin exhaling as the arms descend toward the body again. While the hands descend, your body will begin to turn to the left. The right arm will swing in front of the torso, the left arm will swing behind the torso, and both hands will be facing up (the second photo shows this action from the side). Keep the knees facing forward and turn your body into the crease of the thigh. Avoid overextending by leaning out over the left knee and hip. As you reach out in both directions, use your intention and eyesight to visualize yourself discharging qi from the hands off into the distance.

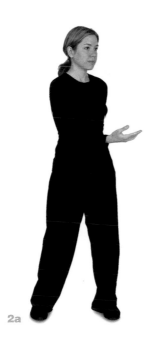

2a

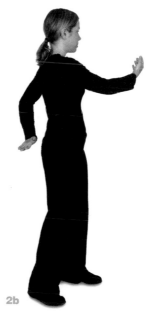

2b

(continued)

Counter Swing *(continued)*

3 Switch to an inhalation and return to the beginning position with arms raised. Be sure to bring your body in complete alignment facing forward before switching to exhalation to the right.

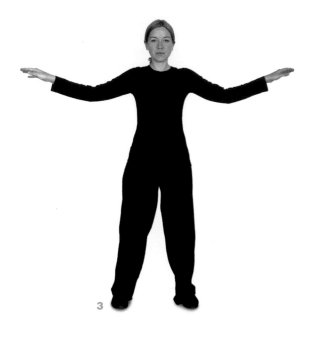

4 As you exhale and drop your arms, begin to turn to the other side. This time the left hand comes in front and the right arm goes behind. Repeat 18 times, alternating left and right sides for a total of 18 "drops" to each side.

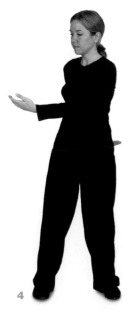

Dropping Post

Dropping Post is a great clearing that gets qi moving through the bones. Consistent with its name, the body mimics the pounding effect of dropping a post onto the ground. The impact of the post hitting the ground shakes off any loose debris that is stuck to it. The tapping action of the heels sends a vibration through the entire body, enabling the release of qi from deep within the core. Dropping Post has an additional benefit for the bones in that the vibration also shakes the bones, sending the signal to the bones to create bone mass. Greater bone density means stronger bones, making this exercise a great way to help address osteoporosis. One repetition of Dropping Post is about 12 times tapping and three times dropping, and one set consists of three repetitions.

1 **From the beginning posture, shorten the stance just enough so that you are comfortable coming up onto your toes. Bend your knees a little more than usual so that they become springlike and you are able to bounce. From this posture, begin to tap the heels to the ground at a comfortable pace. Keep the knees bent and allow them to bend and flex to absorb the impact. Visualize the entire body being soft and supple; allow the limbs to relax and breath. Each time you tap, visualize big chunks of turbid qi being released from your body and draining into the Earth. Allow the chunks to be released even from inside the abdomen and chest. The more relaxed you are as you tap, the more effective the release is. Tap for either three breaths or a specific count of 12 to 15 taps.**

2 **Inhale, filling the body from toe to head, at the same time rising and lifting the heels off the ground. Use your hands to maintain balance by pushing the palms facing out behind you.**

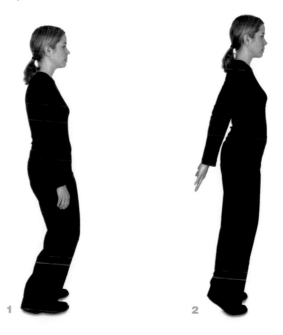

1   2

(continued)

Dropping Post *(continued)*

3 The traditional way to complete this exercise, taught to me by Sifu Johnson, is to rise onto your toes while inhaling and then drop onto a springy platform. After completing the inhalation, switch to an exhalation and let your body drop onto the feet as if you were dropping a post onto the ground. Pretend you're standing on a trampoline so that you keep bouncing up and down. Let the reverberation of the drop keep your body bouncing until you feel the vibration has dissipated. Then, inhale again up onto the toes and drop. Repeat this motion three times. It is extremely important to allow your body to bounce when contacting the Earth. *Do not* tighten the muscles at the knees or lower back. Keep the knees parallel with each other and avoid sinking into the center.

The second way to end this exercise is gentler on the lower back and knees and is better suited for people who have weak knee ligaments and tendons, back injuries, or compromised balance. If you are unsure about which version to practice, start with this version and then work up to the traditional version. Instead of dropping and bouncing when you have inhaled and are on your toes, simply bring your body weight down gently onto the heels, lifting the arms out in front of you (as in a squat). This version of the exercise requires greater emphasis on the focused intention of releasing as you exhale and descend instead of relying on the impact of the heels on the ground.

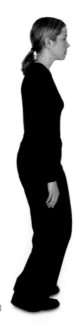

3

Trembling Horse

Have you ever seen a horse shake and ripple its skin to remove flies and other pests? This exercise uses the same principle of shaking and vibration to dislodge and release any turbid or stagnant qi. By shaking each joint in order, a cumulative effect is created that moves qi out from the depths of tissues and sinews and up to the surface where it can be cleansed. The path of the vibration will flow from one extremity to the other and will start as a deep, slow shake, evolving into a quicker, more superficial tremble. Trembling Horse can be repeated three times.

Although this exercise looks funny to the observer, the person doing it feels really great afterward! Many of my students love this exercise so much that we usually add one last repetition of Trembling Horse, free-form style. This means no rules—just shake and let it all go! It's usually followed by plenty of satisfied smiles.

1 Start in the beginning posture. Use natural breathing throughout this part of the exercise. Bring your awareness to your hands. Staying as relaxed as possible, begin to shake the hands, activating the palms and wrists.

2 You'll begin to feel the muscles and joints open and relax. When you feel the wrists are loose, move up to the elbow. Continue to visualize any turbid or stagnant qi being shaken and dislodged from deep within the marrow of the bones, the joints, and the muscles. Guide the vibration up to the shoulders. As you activate each new section, keep the previous section moving. Try not to isolate any section, because the overall movement supports the releasing process.

3 From the shoulders, the shaking descends into the hips. The hips initiate a shimmying motion that guides the ripples of qi down the legs to finally be grounded into the Earth.

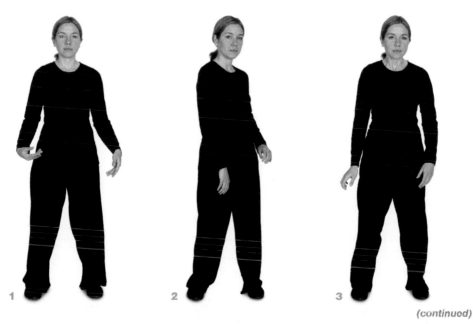

1   2   3

(continued)

Trembling Horse *(continued)*

VARIATION

This exercise can also be performed following the reverse path, from the feet to the hands. It has more of an ascending action with the qi, so people with high blood pressure or who are overactive should avoid this path.

To practice Trembling Horse from feet to hands, activate the action by shaking the feet from side to side (left to right). It will feel a little strange since the feet are firm on the ground. The next step is to guide the shaking up into the ankles and then up the legs to the knees. Keep going through each joint until you reach the shoulders. Then guide the qi down the arms with a rapid shimmying motion, supporting the feeling of release by exhaling and using your intention to guide the turbid qi into the Earth.

This version of the exercise can also be repeated three times.

Cultivation

Cultivation refers to the process of accumulating, refining, or storing qi. This is the main reason we begin working with qigong. By the time you're ready to begin cultivating qi, all three dantian should be activated and qi flow throughout the meridians stimulated. Your body should feel more open, relaxed, and loose.

While the previous sections had the intention of creating a connection between Heaven and Earth, or clearing away turbid qi, this section works with more targeted areas or practices, such as tonifying or purging specific organs, or activating and energizing specific meridians. The stage of cultivation is where qigong achieves a more profound effect and can be considered the section where the focus of your practice lies. It is the part of our routine where our intention shifts from preparing to work to actually doing the work. In addition, the qigong practiced during the cultivating section should be focused toward achieving the goal initially set for practice.

The particular qigong you choose for this portion of the routine will depend on the purpose or goal of your practice. It can be a single qigong movement or a complete set. There are many options to choose from—remember that there are hundreds of styles of qigong. The type of qigong you choose will depend on the focus and intention of your practice. Some options to look at in qigong for health include purging, organ strengthening, relaxing, and tonifying (adding qi). Remember the three applications or categories of qigong: martial, medical, and spiritual. Take time to explore a variety of options and discover all that qigong has to offer. Chapters 6 through 9 describe two preset flows and a few individual qigong exercises that cover qigong for health, qigong for strength, and qigong for relaxation. More information on the benefits of each will be covered in the appropriate chapter.

Centering

After completing your qigong cultivation and before closing your practice, it's a good idea to help your qi settle or root. The centering section is equally important as the clearing section. During the centering, the focus returns to the Taiji Pole and balancing qi, returning qi to the three dantian, and stabilizing any movement that was initiated. Centering is also described as calming, and it invokes the feeling of grounding and relaxing. By the time we reach this phase, the heart rate has elevated, the breathing rate has increased, and the overall qi flow is increased, open, and expanded. This section allows the body to cool down and return qi to any appropriate energetic centers, such as the dantians or organs. Some good centering and balancing exercises are shown in chapter 9.

Closing

The closing is similar to the opening. It is a simple moment when we create a physical, energetic, and mental separation from practicing qigong and returning to our normal activities. There are several ways to perform a closing, but as mentioned in the opening section, the one I use the most is Pulling Down Heavens. The movements are the same as described in the opening on page 42; however, the intention (mind) shifts from establishing a connection to the Earth and Heaven to closing that connection. Although we never completely disconnect from the universal qi, performing Pulling Down Heavens as a closing provides a clear physical, energetic, and mental ending. Since the intention changes in this version of Pulling Down Heavens, let's look at what your closing visualization might be.

Pulling Down Heavens—Step 1

Visualize a silver column of light shining down onto the crown of your head. As you inhale, reach over your head and bring down the column of light over the front of your body like a cool rain, washing over the surface of your skin, removing any turbid qi that might have come to the surface, and releasing it into the ground. Let the cool silver rain rinse the face, chest, abdomen, front of the legs, and tops of the feet all the way down into the ground.

Pulling Down Heavens—Step 2

Visualize a golden column of light shining down onto your crown. As you inhale, reach over your head and bring down the column of light over the back of your body and let it descend like warm oil over the surface of your skin, removing any turbid qi that might have come to the surface and releasing it into the ground. Let the warm golden oil rinse down the back of your head, shoulders, back, glutes, thighs, calves, and heels all the way down into the ground.

Pulling Down Heavens—Step 3

Visualize a white column of light shining over your crown. As you inhale, reach over your head and bring the column of light down the center of your body, connecting through all three dantian and rooting it into the lower dantian. Hold your hands over the lower dantian, actually resting on the skin. Take three deep breaths into the lower dantian, allowing the lower belly to expand as you inhale and contract as you exhale. On the last breath, allow the hands to descend and come to your sides, palms facing the Earth. Hold this posture as long as you like, and when you're ready, step out of the ending posture.

After having completed all the exercises contained within the opening and clearing, you should already feel many changes in your body. You may notice vibration, tingling, or hot and cold spots, maybe even little muscle spasms. Don't worry, all of this is normal and should pass within minutes. These sensations are an indication that qi is flowing to those areas. Increased qi flow stimulates the nerve endings and increases heat, causing the sensations described above. In the case of muscle spasms, it may be the body releasing charges that have been stored in that area for a length of time. In all cases, these symptoms should manifest for a very short time. If for some reason they seem to persist, please contact a qualified qigong instructor or an acupuncturist for advice.

With all the elements of good structure both in posture and in the sequence of a complete qigong routine explained and practiced, it's time to start working with cultivation. The next two chapters outline two qigong sets that are targeted for more specific and in depth work. The Daoist Five focuses more on specific organs, while the Eight Silk Brocade is more of a stretching exercise that works on muscles, tendons, and meridians. It's a good idea to choose either the Daoist Five or the Eight Silk Brocade and avoid doing both back to back until you build proficiency at qigong. Both of these sets provide an excellent workout and will compliment the rest of your qigong routine.

Chapter 6

Qigong for Internal Organ Strength

The Daoist Five qigong set is best suited for maintaining internal organ health. It is based on the wisdom of the Five Elements, which we learned about in chapter 4. Keeping in mind that the elements correspond to specific yin and yang organs, this set of powerful qigong movements restores yin and yang energetic balance, promoting efficient and continuous qi flow from one organ to the next. This set has five individual movements, each of which addresses a particular element.

As we learned in chapter 4, each element represents a specific organ. This means that each of the five movements in the Daoist Five works on both an element and an organ at the same time, where the element is represented by the organ and vice versa. By individually addressing each element and its corresponding organ, the Daoist Five recognizes that the health of our organs is as important as the health of our muscles and bones and that it is important to keep them clear, strong, and flowing with qi. Each movement in the qigong form is designed to stretch the meridians and activate jing, qi, and shen circulation in addition to massaging the internal organs. This qigong form is appreciated for its ability to get straight to the point, and its targeted practice provides immediate results. The exercises can be practiced as a complete flow or individually to address specific organ conditions.

Maintaining Energetic Balance

To get the most benefit out of the Daoist Five, there are a few concepts you may want to consider that can significantly alter your method of practice. Since the purpose of the Daoist Five is to bring the elements back into balance, it is implicitly understood that the current state of any element can be out of balance. The relationship possibilities between the qualities of yin and yang qi in an organ are as follows: deficient (not enough qi), excess (too much qi), or balanced. Therefore, while practicing the Daoist Five, our focus in each element could be to *tonify*, which means increasing the qi level to resolve a deficiency, or to *purge*, which means decreasing qi to resolve an excess. Factors that contribute to organ deficiencies and excesses are

- ► all foods and supplements, medications, and recreational drugs;
- ► thoughts and emotional patterns;
- ► environmental influences, including air and water toxins, radiation, and so on;
- ► lifestyle choices, such as physical activity, sleep patterns, and so on;
- ► medical conditions; and
- ► genetic predisposition.

The focus can also be to *regulate* qi, or support a qi level that is already balanced. Depending on the focus you choose, there will be shifts in your intention and breathing. Let's look at each focus individually to gain a better perspective on what it entails.

Tonify

Tonifying is the action of strengthening, bringing in, or adding things that benefit us or make us stronger. We can tonify emotions, thoughts, behaviors, and the body with focused intention and practices that support tonification on all three levels: jing, qi, and shen. Some examples of tonifying on a physical level include observing a healthy diet and taking herbal supplements. On a psychological or emotional level, tonifying can be done via positive affirmations or cultivating virtues such as kindness, trust, and integrity. Spiritual tonification can include prayer, meditation, and devotional practices. While practicing the Daoist Five Yin qigong, which you will learn about in the next section, tonifying is supported by focusing on inhaling and visualizing healthy qi entering the body. The organ most commonly in need of tonifying is the Kidneys (Water element).

Purge

Purging is the action of releasing and eliminating anything that no longer serves us. We can purge emotions, thoughts, toxins, behaviors, and more with focused intention and practices that support purging on all three levels: jing, qi, and shen.

Some examples of purging on a physical level are herbal cleanses and washes, sweating in saunas or steam baths, and fasting. On an emotional level, purging can be accomplished via therapy or counseling or via emotional expression such as crying, shouting, and laughing. In a spiritual sense, purging can be done through prayers for forgiveness or visualizing yourself covered in divine white light coming from a spiritual source. While practicing the Daoist Five Yin, purging is supported by exhaling and visualizing turbid qi leaving the body. The organ most commonly in need of purging is the Liver (Wood element).

Regulate

Regulating is the action of balancing. We can regulate emotions, thoughts, behaviors, the body, and more with focused intention and practices that support regulation on all three levels: jing, qi, and shen. Examples of regulating include selecting a proper diet according to one's constitution and physical needs, adopting a mindfulness practice that provides constant feedback regarding one's emotions and thought patterns, being conscious of lifestyle choices, and following a regularly defined spiritual practice. However, more often than not we are purging or tonifying while trying to restore balance. While practicing the Daoist Five Yin, which you will learn about in the next section, regulating is supported via equal distribution of attention on inhaling and exhaling as well as balanced intention on the corresponding visualizations of healthy qi entering the body and turbid qi exiting the body.

Several ideas of how to apply the concepts of purging and tonifying to the Daoist Five are included in table 6.1. Each column shows ways to support the intention of purging or tonifying. Remember to choose only one column at a time while working through the Daoist Five qigong set (i.e., don't try to purge and tonify at the same time). You can change the intention the next time you practice. These are just some of the methods and visualizations that are possible. For additional ideas, see figure 4.1 of the Five Elements cycle included in chapter 4.

Remember that it's not necessary to practice all of the concepts included in the table at once; it's better to explore the feeling and benefit of each one individually. Consistency goes a long way when cultivating qi. For example, if you decide to work on purging a particular element, then stay with purging throughout all the elements. The next time you practice, you can change the intention to tonifying or regulating if you want to try a different focus.

Looking at the table, it's easy to see how changing the intention will make a big difference on the effect of the qigong practice, and it highlights the importance of harmonizing the mind or intention with your practice. With all the options we've explored, we can appreciate that although the Daoist Five set has six basic movements, changing the intention to purging, tonifying, or regulating multiplies the practice into many more qigong possibilities. This profound understanding gives you a tool that can be used over and over without exhausting its potential.

TABLE 6.1

Balancing Internal Organ Qi With the Five Elements

	Purge	Tonify
	Focus on exhaling and releasing.	*Focus on inhaling and strengthening.*
Metal/ Lungs	▶ Release grief and sorrow. ▶ Make the "sh" sound while exhaling.	▶ Focus on the virtue of integrity. ▶ Bring in white light or air.
Water/ Kidneys	▶ Release fear. ▶ Make the "chree" sound while exhaling.	▶ Focus on the virtue of wisdom. ▶ Bring in dark-blue water.
Wood/ Liver	▶ Release anger and irritability. ▶ Make the "shu" sound while exhaling.	▶ Focus on the virtue of kindness. ▶ Bring in blue-green young plants.
Fire/ Heart	▶ Release anxiety and overexcitement. ▶ Make the "ha" sound while exhaling.	▶ Focus on the virtue of unconditional love. ▶ Bring in pink or red fire.
Earth/ Spleen	▶ Release worry. ▶ Make the "who" sound while exhaling.	▶ Focus on the virtue of trust. ▶ Bring in yellow-brown earth.

Daoist Five

The Daoist Five has two sections, one that addresses the yang energy of each element and one that addresses the yin energy of each element. The yang energy is addressed first and corresponds to the organs in charge of transforming and transporting nutrients into qi and Blood. Because their functions are digestion and movement, these organs are activated simultaneously in one single exercise, Swaying, which is described next. The yin energy corresponds to the function of regulating and storing qi and is addressed in a separate section where attention is placed on each element and organ individually.

Section I: Daoist Five Yang

We begin with the yang section to activate the meridians along the outside of the arms and legs, the back of the body, and the internal organs related to the digestive system. The purpose of the Daoist Five Yang is to activate the yang organs and meridians. Its pumping action mimics and supports peristalsis, the natural expanding and contracting motion of the digestive system, which increases qi and Blood circulation to the organs and further facilitates its function of transporting and eliminating. Because of the attention the Daoist Five Yang pays to the digestive system, it is an excellent remedy for disorders of the organs of the abdomen and digestion.

The exercise requires rhythmic and coordinated pumping action of the breath, abdomen, and hands, so it may take several repetitions before it becomes a coordinated movement. Try to build a continuous, smooth rhythm that flows effortlessly between each step. The exercise should be performed for 36 repetitions at the very least because it takes time for the rhythm to develop and the body to adjust. Ideally, one can build up to more repetitions, around 250 or more, depending on individual need. If it's too much to keep track of counting while doing many repetitions, just time yourself and keep your practice to less than five minutes. Also, it's best not to practice the Daoist Five Yang with a full stomach, so be sure to allow enough time after a meal for your digestion to settle down. Keep in mind that a normal side effect is belching and passing gas. Just let the air out—it's a great confirmation that the exercise is working!

Swaying

1 **Start in the beginning posture. Bring your hands up to your shoulders by bending at the elbows, palms facing forward, wrists relaxed. Inhale and allow the belly to expand as it fills with breath, filling the organs and meridians with qi. This is the fullest part of the expansion, and I often describe it as *bird belly*—full, round, and tilted forward. You can move the tailbone (tip of the coccyx) back just a little to help the expansion. Visualize the entire body relaxed and full of qi. Visualize the inhalation bringing breath and clean, healthy qi into the entire digestive tract, filling every organ with vitality.**

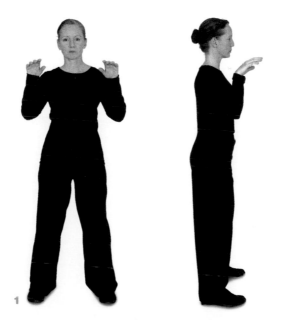

(continued)

Swaying (continued)

2 Begin to exhale and let the hands push forward from the shoulders as though they are beginning to trace the top part of a circle or a ball. When the hands are about a foot (30 cm) away from the shoulders, let them drop or sway all the way down and back behind your hips, making a half circle. Contract the lower abdominal muscles, bringing the belly back in and pushing back softly with the palms. Exhale as soon as the hands begin to move away from the shoulders and end when the hands are pushing behind you. The effort from the muscles in the arms should be minimal; avoid too much tension. When your hands are pushing down on the exhalation, visualize the toxic qi or sludge being released and dispersed into the Earth. This squeezing action supports the natural contraction of the digestive system (peristalsis).

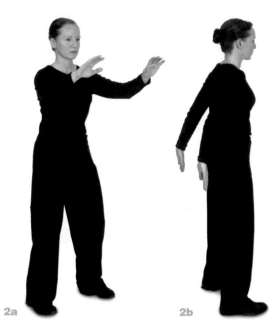

2a   2b

3 Once your hands softly push behind you, inhale and allow them to naturally swing back to the shoulders by bending at the elbows, keeping the palms facing forward. As you inhale and return the hands to the starting position, visualize the palms pulling in qi, filling all the yin meridians and the belly. This completes one repetition.

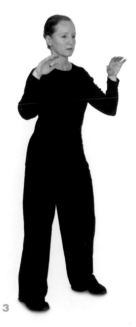

3

Section II: Daoist Five Yin

Once the body has been prepared with the Daoist Five Yang, it's time to go deeper into each specific meridian via the Daoist Five Yin. The Daoist Five Yin addresses each element individually, allowing for deeper exploration into the quality of each organ and more effective purging, tonifying, or regulating of each organ. Although these exercises can be practiced individually, they provide the greatest benefit when practiced as a complete set. The qigong developed for each element is designed to enhance the circulation of jing, qi, shen, and Blood for that element by accessing the corresponding organs. The qigong set begins with the Metal element and moves through the creation cycle in order: Metal, Water, Wood, Fire, and Earth.

Metal

The following movement stretches and contracts the Lung and Large Intestine organs and meridians, further facilitating an exchange of Metal qi. The deep breathing also activates the diaphragm, which further supports peristalsis and the function of the Large Intestine to transport and eliminate. This movement is reminiscent of the action of a bellows (or an accordion) in that it stretches and contracts the space between the arms and lungs. One inhalation and expansion with one exhalation and contraction constitute one repetition. Repeat the exercise for at least nine repetitions. You may increase the repetitions if you desire additional attention on the Metal element.

1 **Start in the beginning posture. Lift your arms straight out in front of you, palms down. Keep the elbows bent and pointing toward the floor, and drop the shoulders and keep them relaxed throughout the entire movement. Keeping the arms parallel to the floor, inhale and begin to move the hands to the sides until they are about 45 degrees to each side. The inhalation matches the opening movement so that the inhalation begins with the arms straight in front and ends when the arms are at 45 degrees. Visualize the arms as the handles of a bellows instrument, opening and expanding, pulling air into the pouch. Visualize the lungs filling with healthy Metal qi by visualizing a white mist in front of you. As you inhale, bring in the white mist to fill the Lung organ and meridians. This completes the first half of the exercise.**

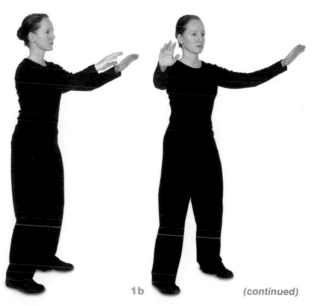

1a   1b   (continued)

Metal *(continued)*

2 Keeping the arms parallel to the floor, turn the palms up and begin to exhale while bringing the arms back to the center. End with palms facing up and arms extended straight ahead of you (keeping elbows and shoulders relaxed). Do not let the hands touch when they reach the center. The exhalation matches the closing movement so that the exhalation begins when the arms are at 45 degrees and ends when the arms are extended straight ahead. Visualize the arms as the handles of the bellows, closing and contracting, releasing air from the pouch. Visualize turbid Metal qi (in the form of grief, illness, or other) being released from your body with the exhalation in the form of a gray mist. This completes the second half of the exercise.

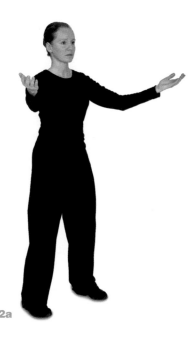

2a

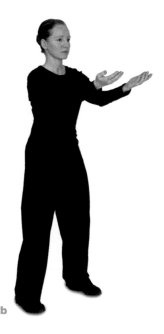

2b

Water

The following movement stretches and contracts the Kidney and Urinary Bladder organs and meridians, further facilitating the exchange of Water qi. The movement mimics the dipping motion of a waterwheel, further supporting the visualization of collecting and storing water. To help understand the motion, visualize yourself as a large waterwheel with a river running in front of your feet, both of which are on the same side of the river. Your arms will turn like the waterwheel, scooping up clear water and releasing turbid water, first in one direction and then the other.

1 Start in the beginning posture and shift your weight to the left leg. Make sure the hip joint is over the knees, which are over the ankles; this ensures a stable foundation and also avoids injuries caused by overextending. Keeping the left knee pointed forward, turn your body toward the left. This creates a crease at the hip joint on the left and extends the right side of the body. Your chest should now be facing about 45 degrees to the left. Wrap the left hand behind the back and let it rest on the right kidney area. If your wrists are flexible enough, you can place the left palm over the right kidney; if not, it's OK to let the palm face away from you. The right arm curls in front of your chest with the hand occupying the same 45-degree angle that the chest is facing. The palm is toward you at eye level so that you're gazing into the center of the palm of your hand (the second photo shows this position from the back).

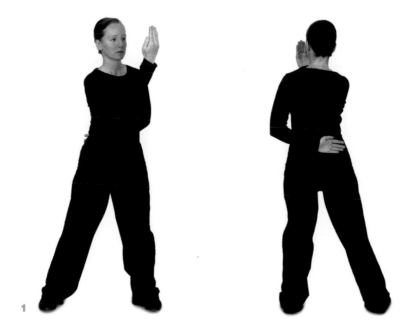

1

(continued)

Water *(continued)*

2 The next step is to begin moving from the left to the right. Begin by moving your weight back to the center while at the same time turning your right palm away from your body. As the body shifts weight from left to right, the hand moves in unison. Keep your gaze centered on the back of your hand throughout the entire movement. This motion is similar to painting the sky with your right palm in a sweeping arc from left to right. Continue moving and shifting to the right until your weight is on the right leg and the hip is over the knee, which is over the ankle. The movement finishes with the body folded into the right hip and the right hand reaching about 45 degrees to the right. The breath matches the movement so that the exhalation begins with your palm at 45 degrees left and ends after you guide the hand to 45 degrees right. Keeping the visualization of the waterwheel, this movement would be tracing the top portion of the wheel. On the exhalation, visualize fear and turbid qi from the Kidneys being released from the palm.

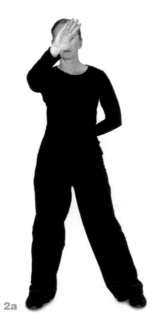

2a

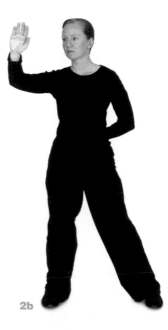

2b

3 Now that the body is in alignment on the right side, begin to turn the tips of the fingers down toward the ground, palm facing the body as if you were about to scoop something. While exhaling, bend at the waist, reach down with your right hand, and guide it from right to left in front of your feet. When the right hand reaches the front of the left foot, your torso will be almost 45 degrees to the left side again. Begin to rise, keeping the arm in a scooping motion, palm up. Inhale while bending and scooping. This completes one circle; repeat for nine circles. Returning to the visualization of the waterwheel, you should feel as though your hand has scooped up water and is carrying it as you rise, returning to the starting point.

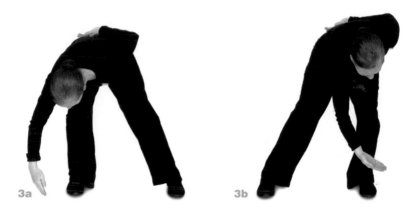

3a   3b

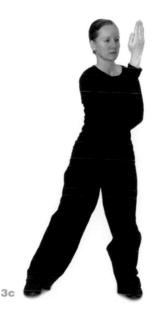

3c

(continued)

Water *(continued)*

4 Once you have completed nine clockwise circles, repeat for nine counterclock-wise rotations. To switch sides, perform this transition: Upon reaching the starting point after nine circles, begin to unwind the left hand from behind the back, bringing it to the front in the same posture the right hand was in. At the same time, wind the right hand behind the back. Pay attention to keeping both arms moving in unison. Finish the transition when the left hand is 45 degrees to the right and the right hand is behind the back, resting on the kidneys.

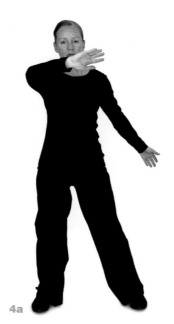

4a

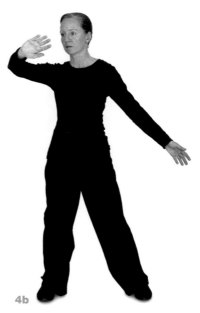

4b

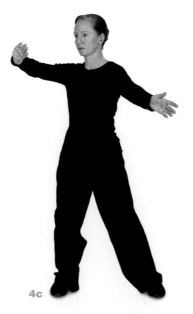

4c

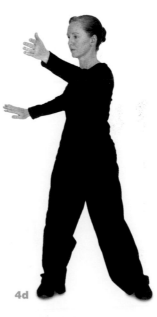

4d

Wood

The following movement stretches and contracts the Liver and Gall Bladder organs and meridians, further facilitating the exchange of Wood qi. The movement mimics the stretching and expanding of a young sapling emerging from a seed as it stretches and reaches forward, leaving its shell behind. It involves pushing and pulling alternating hands while facing directly ahead. Each inhalation charges the body with healthy Wood qi rising from the feet. Each exhalation guides turbid qi out of the feet through the Gall Bladder meridians into the Earth. A good way to feel the energy of this movement is to visualize thick tree sap held between the palms. With each extension and contraction of the palms, the tree syrup is stretched and contracted. The hand that extends has the feeling of pushing, and the hand that contracts has the feeling of pulling. Each of these happens simultaneously so that the overall feeling between the palms is of stretching the tree sap.

1 **Begin with the right arm extended straight in front with the palm facing forward. Keep the shoulder relaxed and the elbow slightly bent. The left hand rests at the left hip, palm up. Exhale in preparation for the next step.**

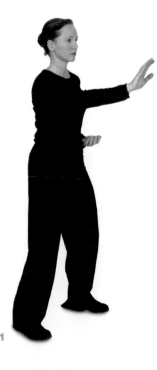

(continued)

Wood *(continued)*

2 Turn both palms clockwise so that the right palm is facing up and the left palm is facing down. Inhale and push the left hand out while simultaneously retracting the right hand to the hip. This step simply reverses the beginning posture. Note that the hands pass one over the other (one palm up, one palm down) at about half the distance in length from the hip to the fully extended arm. When the hands cross each other, the pushing palm slides over the retracting palm without actually touching it.

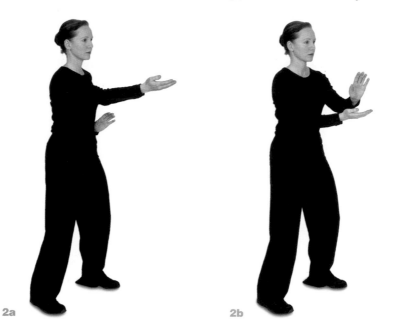

2a   2b

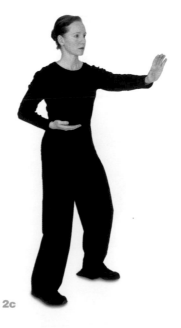

2c

3 Exhale, turn the palms counterclockwise, and retract the left hand while pushing out with the right hand following the same guidelines as in step 2. Coordinate the movement of the arms with the same action in the hips. In other words, each side of the hips will also roll forward or backward on the same side as the hand that extends so that if the right hand is forward, the right hip is forward. The pumping action of the hips activates the Liver and Gall Bladder meridians that run up and down the legs.

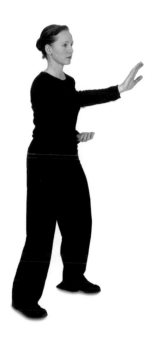

3

Fire

The following movement stretches and contracts the Heart and Small Intestine organs and meridians, further facilitating the exchange of Fire qi. The movement mimics the pushing and pulling of the rising and setting sun. The basic movement is the same, repeated to the left and right sides, pushing the sun away as you extend and pulling it in as you return to the middle. Repeat this exercise for nine repetitions, alternating sides.

The Fire exercise is very effective, and people with high blood pressure or heart conditions should focus on pushing toxic qi away from the body. A feeling of serenity and unconditional love should always be present, which relaxes and calms the Heart. In addition, bringing in soft pink or white light (not red) upon inhalation and maintaining a feeling of peace and softness while doing this qigong will avoid adding fuel to the fire.

1 **Start in the beginning posture. Bring your right hand over the left with palms facing each other as if you were embracing a beach ball. Start to turn the ball clockwise by moving the hands in a clockwise motion, which unrolls the left hand and brings the right hand closer to heart level. Lift the left elbow so that the palm begins turning away from the body. Follow the flow until the left hand is above the head, palm facing away from you as if you were blocking the sun from your eyes. At the same time, the right hand rolls down to heart level until it is vertical, facing left and in front of the midline of the chest. The arm movements occur at the same time the torso is moving from straight ahead to 45 degrees to the left. Allow your weight to shift into the left hip, extending the right leg just a little. Exhale while turning and pushing toward the side. The exhalation matches the move so that you begin facing forward and finish at the maximum extension. Emit qi from the palms of the hands away from you, visualizing any turbid qi being expelled into the distance. Visualize the Heart and Small Intestine meridians being stretched and activated and the Heart being purified. Be careful to keep the shoulders dropped and both elbows bent. Avoid overextending the right arm.**

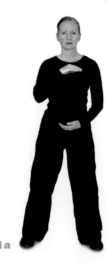

1a

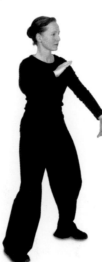

1b

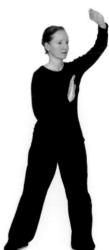

1c

2 Turn the right palm up to catch the ball; the palms should now be facing each other again. Turning the palm is an important step because it switches the position of the palms, setting up the movement to the opposite side. Initiating the motion from your hips, start to return to the beginning posture, pulling the ball back to the center of the chest. The right palm should now be below and the left palm above. Inhale while returning to the beginning position, facing forward. The inhalation matches the movement so that it begins as soon as the hands begin to descend and it ends with the body facing forward and the hands holding the ball in front of the chest. Visualize bringing healthy Fire qi into the body.

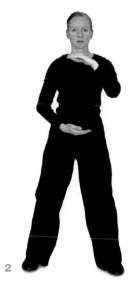

2

3 If done properly, you should now be ready to unwind to the right side, rolling the ball by bringing the left palm down to heart level and the right palm out and above eye level. Turn the left palm up and catch the ball, bringing it back to the center of the chest, facing forward. Exhale while rolling the ball out to the right. Visualize the turbid qi being cleared from the Heart and Small Intestine meridians and organs.

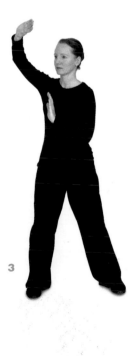

3

Earth

The following movement stretches and contracts the Spleen and Stomach organs and meridians, further facilitating the exchange of Earth qi. The movement mimics the action of the planet Earth spinning beneath the Heavens, the body being the center axis. Repeat this motion for nine repetitions, alternating sides.

People with cervical vertebrae (neck) injuries should not tilt the head backward. The exercise can be performed with the head held upright but with the hands extended over the head. In addition, for those who tend to get dizzy quickly while looking up, reduce the number of repetitions to 3 or 4 and gradually build up to 9 or 12 over time.

1 **Start in the beginning posture and bring your hands together with palms flat, thumbs and index fingers touching each other. (The other three fingers are extended and parallel with the index fingers.) This creates an opening between the index fingers and thumbs that resembles a diamond. Keeping the fingers touching, bring the hands up over the head so that the palms are facing the sky. Tilt your head back so that you can gaze through the opening up into the Heavens. Keep your waist connected to the Earth and the tailbone tilted under. A little clue to help relieve some of the pressure of tilting the head back is to tilt from the top of the neck (around the second and third vertebrae) instead of tilting from the base of the neck at the shoulders. Inhale as the hands make the diamond and rise over the head. Visualize your body as an axis between Heaven and Earth. You will be rotating along that axis, spinning the Earth.**

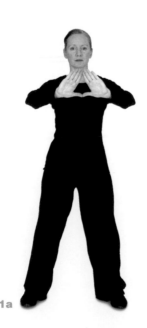

1a

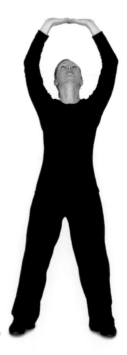

1b

2 While gazing up into the center of the diamond, begin to turn the torso toward the left as far as you can. Be sure to keep the knees facing forward and the hips relaxed.

Coordinate the exhalation with the motion from facing front, finishing at the maximum extension (twist) to the left. When turning to the sides, be sure to keep the tailbone tucked under. It's common to forget and let the pelvis tilt forward, which places extra strain on the waist and can cause injuries. As you twist to the sides, visualize any turbid qi being released from the torso into the Earth through the Stomach meridian.

3 Inhale, bringing the body back to the center, filling the Spleen with healthy Earth qi through the Spleen channel.

4 Exhaling, turn to the right, repeating the same movement but on the opposite side.

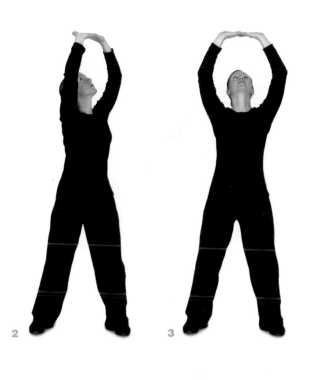

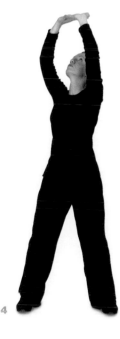

(continued)

Earth *(continued)*

5 After completing the last Earth qigong, return to the center, letting the hands descend down the front of the body while the fingers are touching. Once the hands have reached the lower dantian area, separate the hands and perform three Pulling Down Heavens (see page 42 in chapter 5). This will help you root and regain stability.

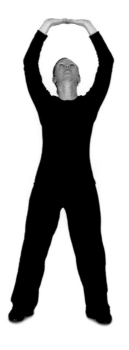

5a

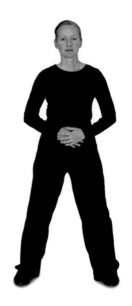

5b

Daoist Five

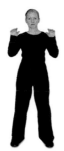
Page 63

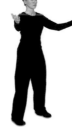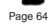
Page 64

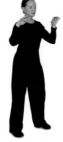
Page 64

Page 64

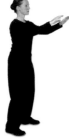
Page 65

Page 65

Page 66

Page 66

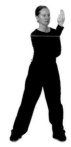
Page 67

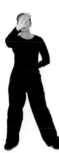
Page 68

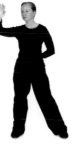
Page 68

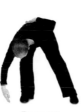
Page 69

Page 69

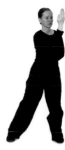
Page 69

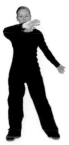
Page 70

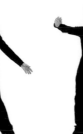
Page 70

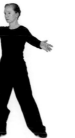
Page 70

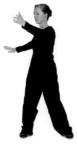
Page 70

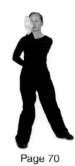
Page 70

(continued)

Daoist Five

(continued)

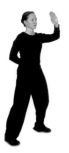

Page 70

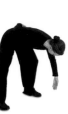

Page 70

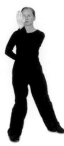

Page 70

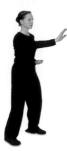

Page 70

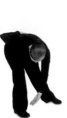

Page 71

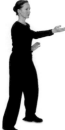

Page 72

Page 72

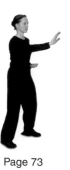

Page 72

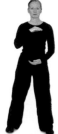

Page 73

Page 74

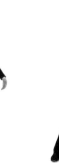

Page 74

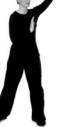

Page 74

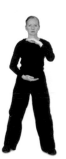

Page 75

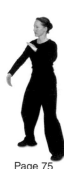

Page 75

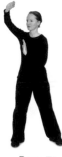

Page 75

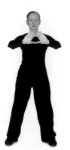

Page 76

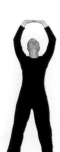

Page 76

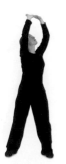

Page 77

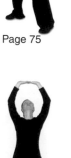

Page 77

Page 77

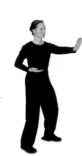

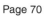

80

Daoist Five

(continued)

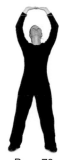

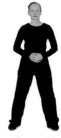

Page 78   Page 78

Chapter 7

Qigong for Optimal Health

The Eight Silk Brocade, also called *Ba Duan Jin*, is a beautiful compilation of eight movements that stretch and relax the tissues and meridians, promoting smooth circulation of qi and Blood throughout the entire body. It is a routine based on slow stretching movements that place more emphasis on how the body moves than other types of qigong, which require focusing on breath control or targeted visualization. The simplicity of the eight movements allows the sequence to be quickly learned and easily practiced.

The origin of the Eight Silk Brocade is hard to determine; however, the most popular theory seems to be that it was created between 1127 and 1279 by General Yue Fei, a famous Chinese general during the Jin Dynasty. As a military leader, he was responsible for preparing troops for battle. All types of people entered his ranks, often arriving in questionable health and with little time to prepare before combat. This inspired General Yue Fei to develop a system of calisthenics that would bring his troops into health and enable them to endure the rigors of primitive conditions; thus, the Eight Silk Brocade was developed.

Throughout its almost 900 years of history, the practice also known as the Eight Section Brocade (and many other variations of that name) has grown to include a seated form and a standing form. Of the two forms, the standing exercise is by far the most popular and has also evolved to include several interpretations of each movement and the advent of Northern and Southern styles. Despite the variations in names, postures, and flows, the basis of the qigong remains the same. It is designed to promote healthy circulation of qi and Blood and improve tendon resilience, internal organ strength, and overall health throughout the entire body. The following pages will present just one of the variations.

Eight Silk Brocade Flow: The Ba Duan Jin Poem

The flow of the Eight Silk Brocade is based on an ancient mnemonic poem passed down from teacher to student for centuries. The poem reminds the practitioner of the nature of the corresponding movements, and each verse invokes key phrases that provide great insight into the benefits of the practice. Recording the qigong set into a poem has helped to maintain its integrity over hundreds of years. The full significance of each verse becomes clear once the actual movements have been learned. The original poem along with an English translation is as follows.

Ba Duan Jin		Eight Silk Brocade
Verse 1	雙手托天理三焦	Double hands hold up Heaven to regulate the Triple Heater
Verse 2	左右開弓似射鵰	Left and right open a bow like shooting a golden eagle
Verse 3	調理脾胃雙臂舉	Regulate the Spleen and Stomach by lifting the arms
Verse 4	五勞七傷向後瞧	Five weaknesses* and seven injuries, turn and look backward
Verse 5	搖頭擺尾去心火	Shake the head and swing the tail to remove Heart Fire
Verse 6	背後七顛百病消	Seven disorders and hundreds of illnesses disappear and are left behind your back
Verse 7	攢拳怒目增氣力	Screw the fist with glaring eyes to increase strength
Verse 8	兩手攀足固腎腰	Both hands pull the feet up, strengthen Kidneys and waist

*The five weaknesses are related to the five yin organs (see chapters 4 and 6).

Eight Silk Brocade

Regular practice of the Eight Silk Brocade improves the circulation of Blood and qi. We know from previous chapters that Blood and qi circulation is important to avoid the onset of disease; when our body is not moving, aches and pains begin to manifest. This qigong set provides a safe way to address the entire body. It stretches and contracts the tendons, making them resilient and supple like silk. Strong tendons enable us to stand up straight, to walk more correctly, and to avoid broken bones or joint injuries. In addition, the movements of the Eight Silk Brocade strengthen the heart, lungs, and digestive system. By bending, twisting, and leaning, it increases the flexibility of the spine and the exchange of cerebrospinal fluid, and this set improves the strength and flexibility of the shoulders and hips. By coming onto the toes, it improves balance and coordination. By moving the eyes and arms, it improves the quality of the brain, allowing for relaxation and clarity of thought. It is a simple method of achieving radiant health inside and out.

The Eight Silk Brocade is best practiced as a complete set. Individual movements can be isolated, but the most benefit is obtained when it is followed from beginning to end. Each movement can be practiced for multiple repetitions, sometimes as many as 24 or 36. However, you should start with three repetitions. You can build up to many more over time, but pace yourself so that it's possible to complete the entire Eight Silk Brocade set. You'll be surprised to see how much benefit you can get out of just three repetitions!

The following pages describe the Eight Silk Brocade practice. Each section starts with the traditional name for the movement. A section is also included that highlights the benefit of each exercise. The description itself is considered one repetition. Note that the breathing pattern in this form is different from the Daoist Five. In this particular set, an inhalation is used when expanding and an exhalation is used when contracting.

First Piece of Silk: Propping Up Heaven

The energetic tapestry of the Eight Silk Brocade is first woven with the strength and stability of the bear. Bears are large, heavy animals with sturdy legs that support their massive structure. Bears stand on their toes to reach for honey and berries and then sink onto their haunches to enjoy the sweetness of the prize. Embody the heaviness and slow stretch of a bear to perform this qigong.

This exercise is commonly acknowledged to benefit the Triple Heater and Pericardium meridians in addition to the Heart and Lung organs. However, the stretching action to each side activates all of the organs of the torso and places some emphasis on the yin channels of the arms. By lifting the arms, qi is stimulated to flow more smoothly between the top and bottom half of the body, counteracting sinking qi and creating a feeling of being lifted. By coming onto the toes, it also improves balance.

1 **Start in the beginning posture with arms and hands relaxed at your sides. The lower half of the body is rooted into the Earth. The upper body remains relaxed and in proper qigong alignment. Begin by bringing the hands together in front of the body, fingers interlaced, palms up. When they are at chest level, turn the palms up toward Heaven. Continue raising the hands until they are over the head. Coordinate the rising action of the hands with lifting your body onto your toes. Just lift your heels off the ground; it is not necessary to come up all the way. Inhale in one long breath as the hands begin to travel upward following the midline of the body. The inhalation, hands, and body fill and lift simultaneously, each ending at the same time. Visualize the breath and arms pulling up qi from the Earth all the way over the head. Use your intention to push up even further.**

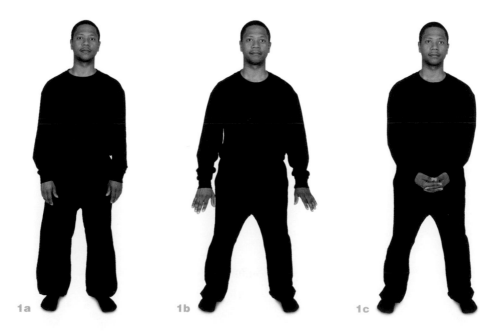

1a   1b   1c

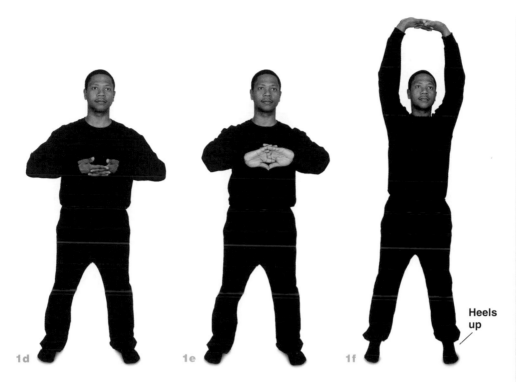

1d 1e 1f

Heels up

2 Keep the hands over the head and begin to exhale and lower your body onto the heels. Return to beginning stance from the waist down. Pay attention to the hips and make sure that your lower dantian is rooted into the Earth and that the tailbone is tucked under. Exhale as you descend from the toes all the way to feet flat on the ground. Visualize yourself sinking back into the Earth and creating a solid foundation that is strong like a bear.

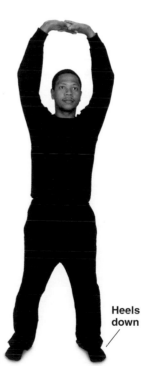

Heels down

2

(continued)

First Piece of Silk: Propping Up Heaven *(continued)*

3 Still facing forward, begin to arch (or lean) the upper body (above the waist) toward the right. The head, shoulders, and hips are all still in vertical alignment. In other words, avoid leaning or bending at the waist. Extend only as far as you feel comfortable; there should be no pain or strain from overextending. Inhale as you extend to the right. Feel your qi coming out the palms of your hands, activating the left side of the body.

4 Exhale and bring your torso back into the middle position.

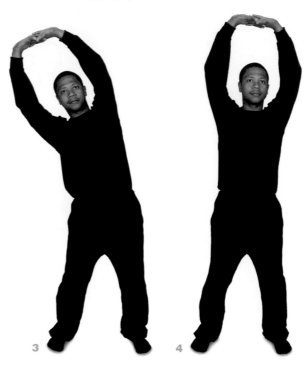

5 Inhale and stretch to the left as described in step 3.

6 Exhale and return to the middle position.

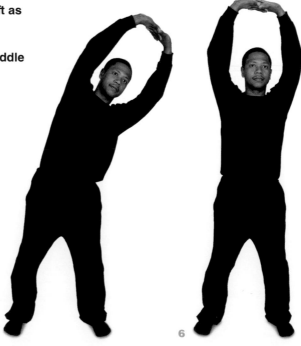

7 Turn the palms down and allow the arms to sink back down to the lower dantian following the midline of the body. Separate the palms and bring the arms to the sides of the body. This completes one repetition.

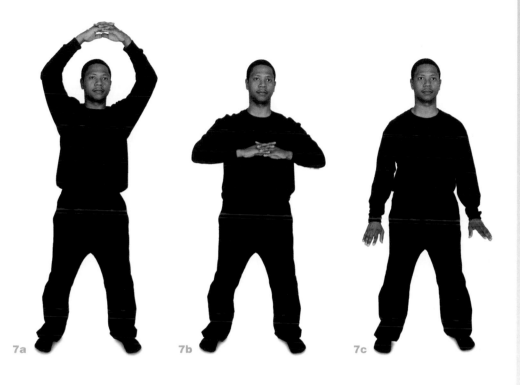

7a   7b   7c

Second Piece of Silk: Drawing the Bow Left and Right

The second piece of brocade is woven with the focus and direction of an archer's arrow. With precision, the archer pulls the bow, aiming for the golden eagle. All the tendons of the arms and shoulders are activated as the archer stretches the bow. Following the tip of the arrow, the archer fixes his gaze on the target and releases the power within. Embody the feeling of being an archer and shoot the arrow left and right.

This exercise strengthens the tendons of the shoulders and elbows, strengthens and relaxes the waist, increases lung capacity, and tonifies the Kidneys.

1 **Start in the beginning posture; you can widen the stance for additional focus on the legs and hips. Bring the hands together, palms up, at the midline of the body. Do not interlace the fingers. The left hand will come up above the right hand. Continue to lift, bringing the hands up to the height of the shoulders. You will need to bend and lift the elbows. With your left hand, grasp the bow by making a fist, palm toward the body. Lift the left elbow as if you were preparing to pull a bow. With the right hand, point the arrow by making an *L* shape with the index finger and thumb. You may also use the index and middle fingers pointed up with the thumb wrapped into the other two closed fingers. Pull with the left hand and extend the right arm, as in shooting an arrow. Elbows are shoulder height, all of which are in alignment. Pull from the back to stretch the bow.**

The breath is one long inhalation that begins when the hands begin to move toward the middle of the body and ends when the arrow has been shot. Feel the qi rising in the torso and expanding laterally at the shoulders.

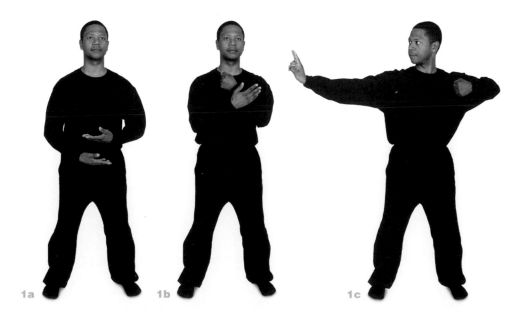

1a   1b   1c

2 Release the arrow by letting the arms contract. Fold the right arm so that the hand is at chest height, next to the left hand. As you exhale, let both hands descend to the beginning posture. Exhale when releasing the arrow all the way down until both hands are by the sides. Visualize the arrow being released and the tendons relaxing. The breath and mind return to the torso and settle in the lower dantian.

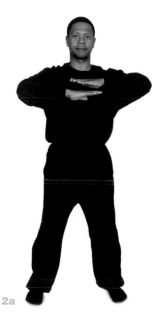

2a

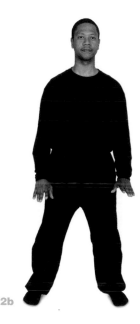

2b

(continued)

Second Piece of Silk: Drawing the Bow Left and Right *(continued)*

3 Repeat steps 1 and 2 on the left side. This concludes one repetition. Repeat to right and left sides for the prescribed number of repetitions.

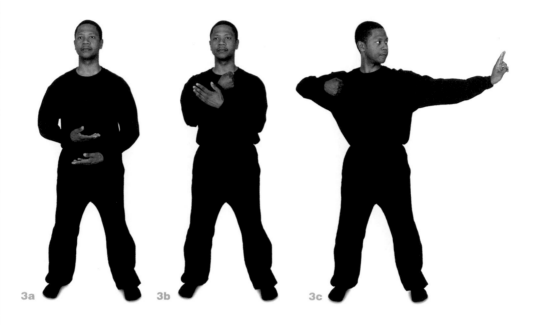

3a   3b   3c

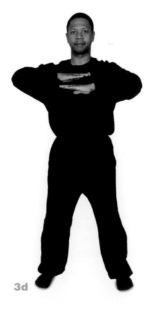

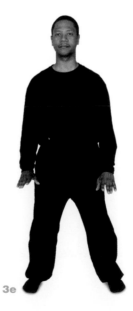

3d   3e

Third Piece of Silk:
Separating Heaven and Earth

The third section of silk is animated in the agility of the monkey. With its long, nimble arms, the monkey is able to swing from limb to limb, switching hands from left to right with ease. That extending, contracting, and switching is brought to life in this piece of the brocade as the monkey weaves his thread up and down, side to side.

This exercise has a clear intention of working with the Spleen and Stomach meridians, which run up and down the legs and torso. The intention of stretching in opposite directions (up and down) clears the digestive system and middle and lower dantian. By turning the wrists, healthy joint articulation in the hands is promoted and can counteract rheumatoid arthritis.

1 **Start in the beginning posture with arms and hands relaxed at your sides. The lower half of the body is rooted into the Earth. Feel the legs connect to the ground and sink the lower dantian into the root. The upper body remains relaxed and in proper qigong alignment. Begin by inhaling and bringing both hands together in front of the body. The fingers do not interlace. Start with the right hand coming up following the midline, keeping the left hand in alignment with the midline but under the right hand. Both palms are up. When both palms reach the height of the stomach, turn the left palm down. The palms will now move in opposite directions: The right palm keeps going up while the left palm goes down. In order for the right palm to ascend, it must turn up. Push from the center of the palms in opposite directions. Keep the elbows slightly bent. The breath is one long inhalation from the beginning of this movement until the palms are extended in opposite directions. Feel the side of the body with the lifted arm stretch and expand. Keep the hips connected to the Earth.**

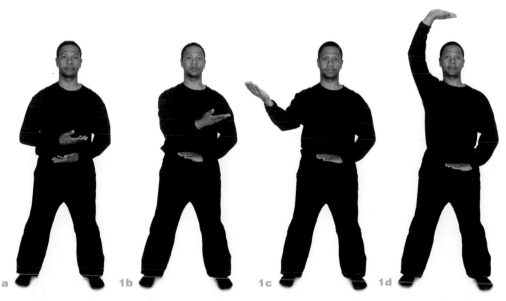

1a   1b   1c   1d

(continued)

Third Piece of Silk: Separating Heaven and Earth (continued)

VARIATION

There is a variation of this movement that further activates the Spleen and Stomach meridians. After the arms are extended in opposite directions and the top hand is over the head, gently turn to the side with the bottom hand to further stretch the extended side. In this particular step, because we started with the right hand, we will stretch to the left.

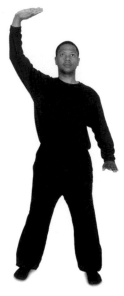

2 Turn the palms to face each other and begin to bring them back to stomach level. Once they are at the same height, turn both palms to face the Earth and guide them back to the beginning posture. The breath is one long exhalation from the maximum expanded posture until both palms are at the beginning posture. Feel the body begin to contract again. Any turbid qi that may have been brought to the surface is expelled into the Earth upon exhaling and pushing down with both palms.

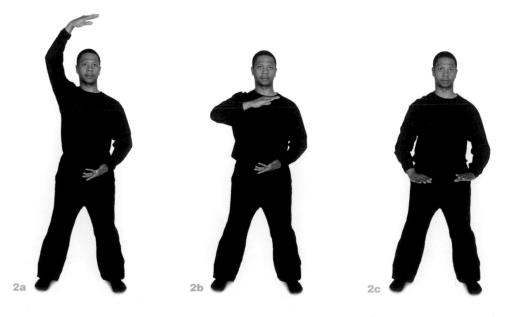

2a   2b   2c

3 Repeat the movement by switching hands and sides. This time the left hand is above the right hand as it rises along the midline of the body. If adding the extra extension, turn to the right.

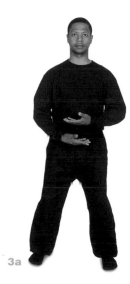

3a

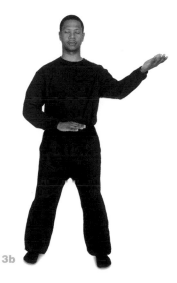

3b

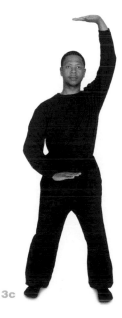

3c

(continued)

Third Piece of Silk: Separating Heaven and Earth *(continued)*

4 Repeat step 2, this time with the left hand descending and the right hand rising until they meet at stomach level. Then turn both palms down and return to beginning posture. This concludes one repetition. Repeat to the right and left sides for the pre-scribed number of repetitions.

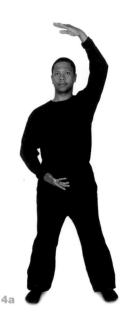
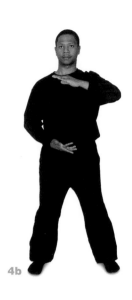
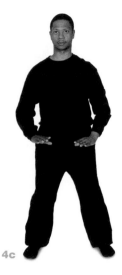

4a   4b   4c

Fourth Piece of Silk: Turning Inner Vision

Drawing in the energy of the fourth piece of brocade, our tapestry now embraces the snake. As the snake peers out of his hiding place, he slowly turns his head from side to side, observing his surroundings. The gentle gaze extends to all directions, first turning his head to the right and then to the left. This is a satisfied snake, free from fear or viciousness, just another of nature's creatures enjoying life.

This exercise strengthens eyes and Liver meridians. It gently stretches the neck, breaking up stagnation in the cervical vertebrae. The soft turn to each side also gently stretches the entire spine and stimulates circulation to the head. This alternating activation of the lateral sides of the head and body improves balance, decreases dizziness, and tonifies the central nervous system. The hands on the waist support the Belt Vessel and Kidneys.

1 **Start in the beginning posture, keeping the hands relaxed by the sides. The movement itself is quite easy. First, slowly turn your head to the right. Once the head has turned comfortably to its maximum point, the eyes follow, looking behind. Avoid overextending; turn only as far as feels comfortable and then turn the eyes. Match the breath to the turning motion so that it feels as if you're turning your head because of the breath. This is one long inhalation. Feel the Liver meridian activate as you turn. This will be accomplished by simply bringing slight awareness to the left foot. Do not visualize qi rising through the leg and into the eyes; just let the energy follow the movement.**

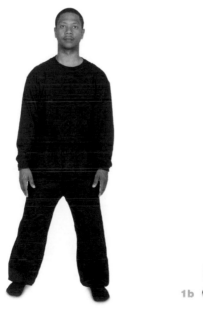
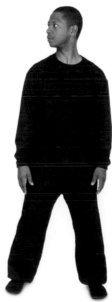

1a   1b

(continued)

Fourth Piece of Silk: Turning Inner Vision *(continued)*

2 Slowly turn the head back to the front. Eyes return to face forward. Match the breath to the movement by exhaling in the same length of time it takes to return to the beginning posture. Feel the body relax, including the eyes and mind.

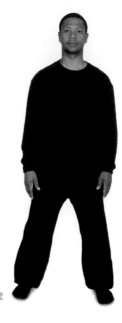

3 Repeat the movement in step 1 to the left. Inhale and turn the head at the same time, extending the eyes softly to the back.

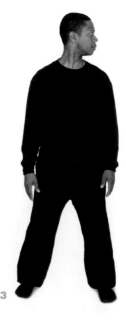

4 Return to face the front. Repeat these four steps for as many repetitions as you are working on in the entire Eight Silk Brocade, and then proceed to the next step.

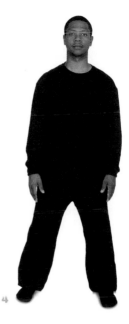

5 Place the hands on the kidneys and continue turning the head and vision side to side for the number of repetitions used in the previous steps. The breath is identical to the first part of the exercise—inhale as you stretch, exhale as you contract. Bring your awareness to the Kidneys, allowing these to also expand and contract according to the exercise.

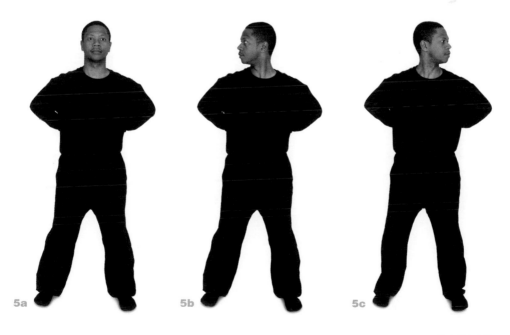

5a   5b   5c

(continued)

Fourth Piece of Silk: Turning Inner Vision *(continued)*

6 The hands come to the front of the body, palms up, as if embracing a large ball. A little clue on how to better feel this part of the exercise is to imagine holding a large load of laundry. Your arms would have to bend at the elbows to grasp it and your back would expand and stretch to allow the arms some room. In addition, the clothes would have weight to them, so the palms and inside of the arms would also be activated.

Slowly turn your head to the right and when the head has turned comfortably to its maximum point, the eyes follow, looking behind. Avoid overextending; turn only as far as feels comfortable and then turn the eyes. The breath is similar to the other steps where you inhale as you stretch, exhale as you contract, but here you match the breath to the turning motion so that it feels as if you're turning your head because of the breath. Bring your awareness to the torso and feel it expand and fill with qi as you inhale and relax as you exhale. Feel the Liver meridian activate as you turn. This will be accomplished by simply bringing slight awareness to the left foot. Do not visualize qi rising through the leg and into the eyes; just let the energy follow the movement. Slowly return your gaze and head until it faces forward. Repeat for as many repetitions as you are practicing in each exercise.

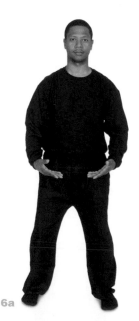

6a

6b

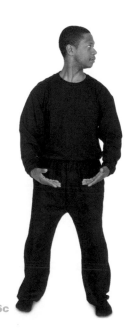

6c

Fifth Piece of Silk: Return to the Source

The dragon weaves the fifth piece of silk into the brocade. Its long, flexible body allows it to roll and turn. Conjuring images of protective scales, the poem teaches us that illnesses slide off our backs like the dragon swimming through the air. The dragon implies rooted feet that firmly grasp the ground and movement above from the waist and arms. The energy of the dragon is of lifting and holding.

This exercise provides flexibility to the spine, creating supple tendons and removing any stagnation. The rising and falling rippling of the spine promotes smooth flow of qi along the Governing Vessel and Conception Vessel. The up-and-down motions strengthen the waist and back and tonify the Kidneys. The downward bend helps to bring qi up into the head, nourishing the brain functions and clearing thoughts. If one is able to touch the floor while bending over, the contact between the hands and the Earth creates a soft circuit excellent for energetic grounding. Finally, stretching the legs stretches the yin meridians of the legs, enabling smooth flow of qi up into the torso.

1 **Start in the beginning posture. Bring the hands together at the midline of the body, palms facing up. Interlace the fingers and bring the hands up to chest height. At this point, turn the palms away from the body and continue lifting the arms so that the palms are facing the sky and the arms are extended. Remember to not lock the elbows. This part is similar to Propping Up Heaven, the first piece of the brocade. The breath is one long inhalation from when you begin to move until the hands are extended over the head. Just relax and feel the body stretch and open.**

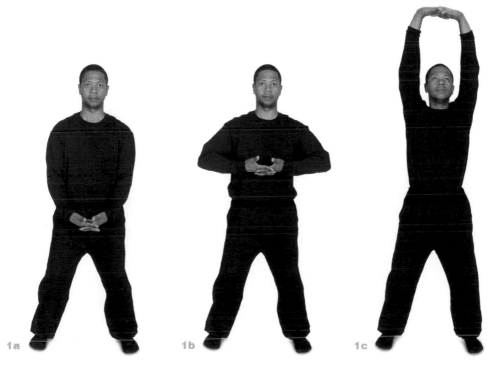

1a   1b   1c

(continued)

Fifth Piece of Silk: Return to the Source (continued)

2 Bending at the hips, reach forward with the hands still interlaced. Bend, fold, and reach as far down to the ground as you can comfortably go. Hold this position for a few seconds. Exhale in one long breath all the way down. Again, relax and feel the body opening, the muscles melting, and the spine becoming fluid.

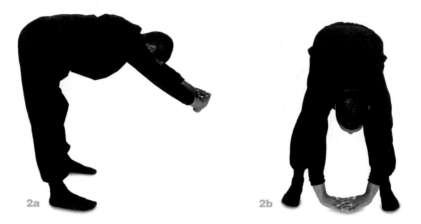

2a

2b

3 Turn the palms up and roll the spine back into the beginning posture by tucking in the hips first and then slowly stacking the vertebrae one on top of the other. After you are standing with the back erect, let the hands come back the sides. Inhale as you rise. Feel the body fill with qi and settle down in the ground again. Repeat these steps for the prescribed repetitions.

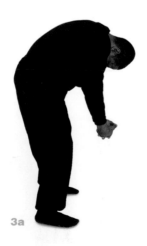

3a

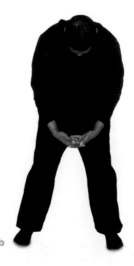

3b

Sixth Piece of Silk: Extinguishing the Fire

The sixth piece of brocade invites us to open our wings like the mythical fenghuang. Regal and auspicious, the Chinese phoenix is full of life and embodies the union of yin and yang. Its enormous size is symbolic of the great virtue it represents. When the fenghuang flies through the sky on the lofty clouds of immortals, turning its mighty plumage left and right, it carries a message of peace and is an omen of good things to come.

This exercise relaxes the Heart by promoting circulation of Kidney (Water) energy. Opening the arms, extending the back, and being in the low stance activate all the yin and yang meridians of the body in both the arms and legs. The exercise strengthens the knees and relaxes the hips. It stretches the spinal column, releasing stagnation and promoting circulation of cerebrospinal fluid.

1 **Start in the beginning posture. Bring your hands onto the tops of the thighs, with the four fingers on the inside of the leg and the thumbs on the outside. Slowly slide your hands down the thighs all the way to the knees. However, instead of bending over at the waist, the hips descend as well so that when you finish, you're in a squatting position. The hips do not descend further than the knees. Keep the elbows bent and the hips low. Curve the back by pushing the sacrum area slightly out.**

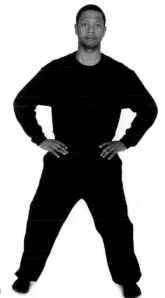

1a

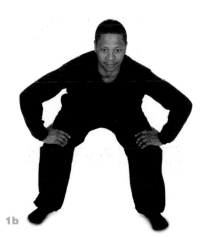

1b

(continued)

Sixth Piece of Silk: Extinguishing the Fire (continued)

2 Push against the left knee with the left hand for stability and turn your torso toward the right. Drop the left shoulder for better alignment and further extension to the right. Turn your head so that you're looking over your shoulder (somewhat up to the sky). The breath is one long inhalation from facing front to looking over the right shoulder. Just relax and feel the entire body expand. This is a difficult exercise, so it's better to avoid active visualizations.

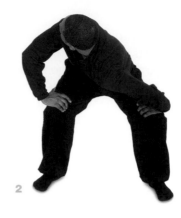

3 Exhale and come back to the center, facing forward. Remain with the hips down. Do not stand up.

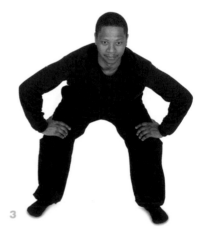

4 Repeat the exercise to the left by pushing with the right hand and dropping the right shoulder. Turn the head to the left and lift the gaze to the sky. Repeat these steps for an equal number of repetitions to each side, remembering to completely center facing forward between each extension. Once you have finished the prescribed number of reptitions to each side, return to beginning posture by rolling the spine, vertebra by vertebra, until you've returned to full standing position.

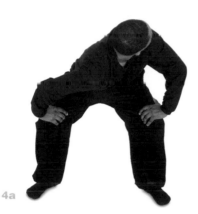

4a

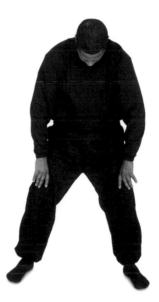

4b

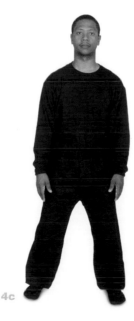

4c

Seventh Piece of Silk: Your Life's Purpose

The mighty lion weaves his strength into the brocade with the seventh piece of silk. Fierce and brave, the lion attacks demons with his deadly paws. Fiery eyes intimidate anyone who dares to challenge the lion, and with his fist he destroys any obstacles in the way. Find your own strength within and express it in your fist as a fearless warrior. The lion is also related to the Heaven trigram, which stands for pure yang and home from which all souls are born. Search Heaven to find your life's purpose.

This exercise benefits the Heart, the central nervous system, and circulation. It counteracts sinking qi and stimulates heat in the body.

1 **Start in the beginning posture. Bring the hands up to the hips and make soft fists. The palm within the fist will be facing up. Next, with your right arm, begin to unwind the fist as the arm extends forward. End with the fist straight ahead (palm down) just under shoulder height. Inhale from the time you begin to unwind the fist until the arm is extended. Use your fierce eyes to send qi out to the fist.**

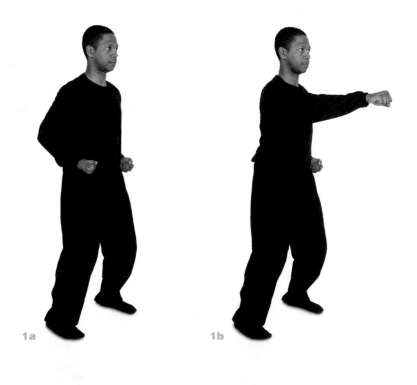

1a   1b

2 Release the punch and open the hand. Turn the hand over so the palm is up and return the hand to the hips with the fist closed. Exhale as you relax the punch and return the palm. Allow the body to relax. Repeat the movement on the left side, extending the left fist and then returning it to the hips. Repeat to alternating sides for the prescribed repetitions.

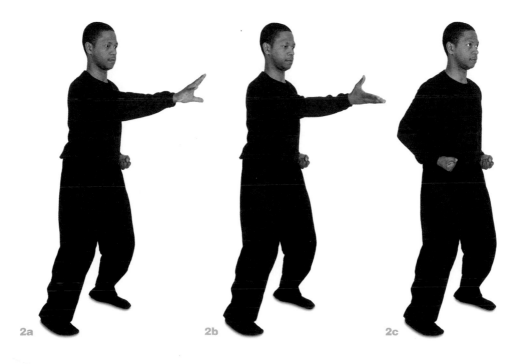

2a   2b   2c

Eighth Piece of Silk: Stimulate Life

The last piece of silk in the brocade is represented by the mythical unicorn (called *qilin* in China). The unicorn is an embodiment of purity and is considered a virtuous animal. It is related to the Earth trigram, and as the final strand of the Eight Silk Brocade, it can be considered the grounding piece. The unicorn takes great care to avoid injuring life and thus is quick and light on its feet. Embody the unicorn to lift your body to purity.

This exercise tonifies the Kidneys, which in turn decreases dizziness. It improves balance by working with the toes and calves. In addition, it stimulates the flow of qi through the Governing and Conception Vessels.

1 **Start in the beginning posture. Keep your hands by your sides and begin to rise onto your toes by lifting the heels off the floor. It is not necessary to rise high onto the toes; work only with what feels comfortable for you. Once you come up onto the toes, lift the chin and look up. You can use your hands for stability by slightly pressing back with them as you rise. Inhale from the beginning until your chin is lifted. Visualize the front of the body expanding and filling with healthy qi.**

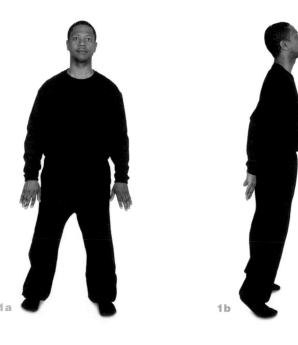

1a   1b

2 Let the chin come down and the eyes return to gaze forward. The heels return to being flat on the ground, and the hands are by your sides again. Exhale as the body relaxes and returns to the beginning posture. Allow the body to relax. Repeat these two steps for the prescribed repetitions.

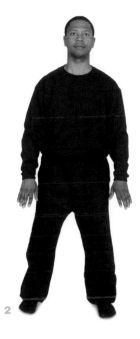

2

3 Bring your hands to rest on the waist, palms facing the kidneys. This posture is identical to the snake. Rise onto the toes and lift the chin. Inhale as you rise. Visualize the front of the body filling and expanding with qi. Keep the hands on the waist and return to beginning posture by placing the heels flat on the floor. Exhale as you descend. Allow the body to relax and sink back into the Earth.

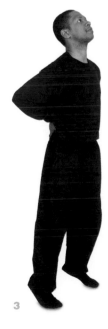

3

(continued)

Eighth Piece of Silk: Stimulate Life (continued)

4 Bring the arms to the front of the body as if you are embracing a large ball. This posture is identical to the last one of the snake. Inhale as you rise. Keep the hands holding the imaginary ball and then return the heels of the feet so they are flat on the floor again. Exhale as you descend. Allow the body to relax and sink back into the Earth. Repeat steps 3 and 4 for the prescribed repetitions.

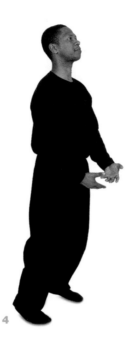

4

Eight Silk Brocade

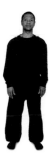
Page 86

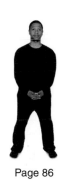
Page 86

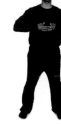
Page 86

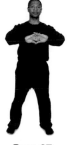
Page 87

Page 87

Page 87

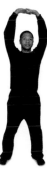
Page 87

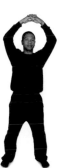
Page 88

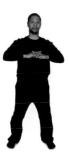
Page 88

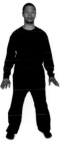
Page 88

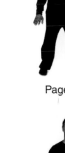

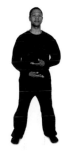
Page 88

Page 88

Page 89

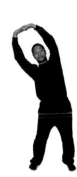
Page 89

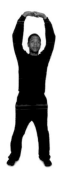
Page 89

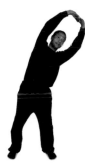
Page 90

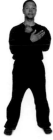
Page 90

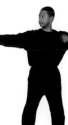
Page 90

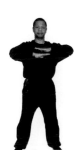
Page 91

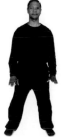
Page 91

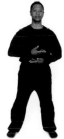

Page 92

(continued)

Eight Silk Brocade

(continued)

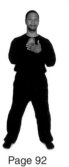

Page 92

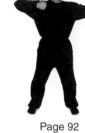

Page 92

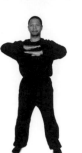

Page 92

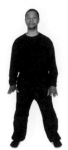

Page 92

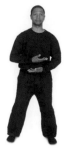

Page 93

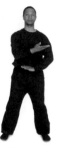

Page 93

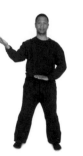

Page 93

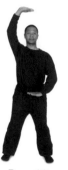

Page 93

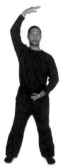

Page 94

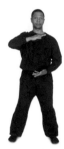

Page 94

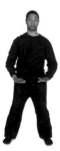

Page 94

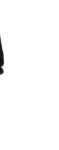

Page 95

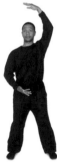

Page 95

Page 95

Page 96

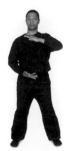

Page 96

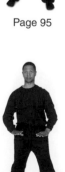

Page 96

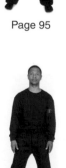

Page 97

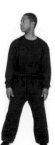

Page 97

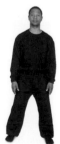

Page 98

Eight Silk Brocade

(continued)

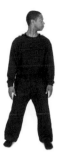

Page 98

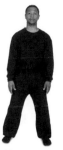

Page 99

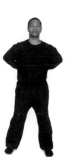

Page 99

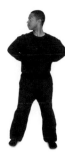

Page 99

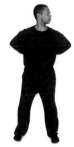

Page 99

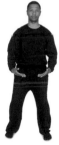

Page 100

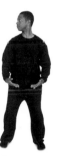

Page 100

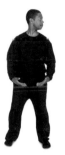

Page 100

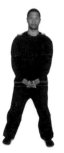

Page 101

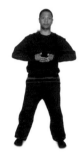

Page 101

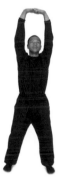

Page 101

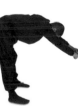

Page 102

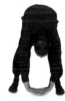

Page 102

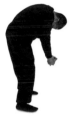

Page 102

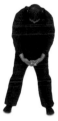

Page 102

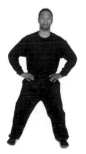

Page 103

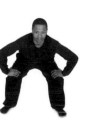

Page 103

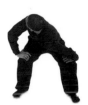

Page 104

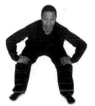

Page 104

Page 105

(continued)

Eight Silk Brocade

(continued)

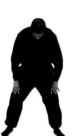

Page 105

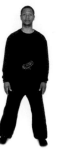

Page 105

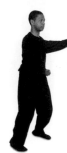

Page 106

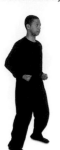

Page 106

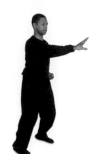

Page 107

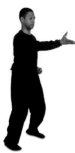

Page 107

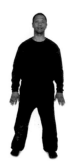

Page 107

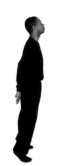

Page 108

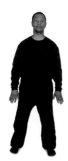

Page 108

Page 109

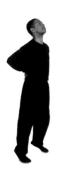

Page 109

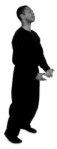

Page 110

Chapter 8

Qigong for Stress Relief

The exercise we will work with as qigong for the relief of stress is Turning and Winding the Belt Vessel. It is a simple and gentle qigong movement based on spinning circles that relaxes yet builds qi at the same time. Of all the qigong forms I've taught, this is by far the most popular. The movement is based on tracing a horizontal circle both clockwise and counterclockwise. The repetition of the circles creates a soothing rhythm that calms the spirit and relaxes the body. In addition, it is an excellent meditation for tonifying the Kidneys and the Belt Vessel as well as stimulating qi flow along the waist.

The Belt Vessel is one of the eight Extraordinary Vessels, a group of special energetic meridians not included in the primary 12 we discussed in chapter 4. The Belt Vessel is located at the waist and runs horizontally like a belt. It is the only horizontal meridian of the body and is considered the linking meridian that connects and distributes energy to all the other vessels. In addition, the Belt Vessel has a deep connection with the Ming Men, or Gate of Life. The Gate of Life is located on the lower back at waist level and is an important qi epicenter that can affect your overall health and vitality. Strong qi flow through the Belt Vessel and Gate of Life creates a full-body energetic cushion that both protects from external influences and boosts the wei qi fields.

Practicing Turning and Winding the Belt Vessel aids in maintaining a healthy Belt Vessel, which in turn can help to avoid conditions such as impaired circulation in the legs, which can cause cramps and numbness; stagnation in the pelvic region, which can lead to many reproductive and elimination disorders; pain and tension in the hips due to inactivity, and pain in the sacrum or lumbar region due to inactivity or qi stagnation. In the second part of the exercise, the Large Circle, activating the eyes assists in supporting qi flow along the Liver and Gall Bladder channels, reducing anger or irritation and improving vision.

Turning and Winding the Belt Vessel relies on the circular movement of energy to stimulate qi flow in specific energetic places. As previously mentioned, working the Belt Vessel is a main part of the exercise; however, the lower dantian is also actively stimulated. The movement of this qigong massages the lower dantian and spins it in the opposite direction of the Belt Vessel. Fortunately, this action occurs spontaneously and does not require active concentration from the practitioner. Therefore, our attention can relax, and we can focus on enjoying the movement and allowing the body to be open and receptive to its natural effects.

Flowing-Seaweed Visualization

Throughout this exercise, mental visualization is not as focused as in other qigong movements. Although the effects are very specific, a relaxed mind is more effective than one that is attempting to create a precise result. Therefore, it is much better to allow the mind to relax and drop into the smooth circular movements and breathing, feeling the qigong rather than visualizing specific energetic patterns or images. The following visualization is designed to do just that. Its purpose is to relax the body and mind and create a safe, soothing environment in which to practice.

Visualize yourself as seaweed at the ocean shore. Your seaweed roots are planted near the beach where the waves rise and retreat on the sand. Relaxed and without any tension, you follow the gentle rising and falling of the swell and waves, first expanding and reaching for the shore, then contracting and returning to depths of the ocean, repeating the timing of the waves in perfect rhythm over and over. Let your body become loose and soft like fresh seaweed without any resistance to the push and pull of the water. Allow the feeling of expanding and contracting to guide you from within so that the movements of your arms and body rise and retreat naturally. All motion is initiated from the center core while the limbs trail behind, flowing in the current. Let the breath fill and empty accordingly, furthering the sensation of opening and closing. Allow the water to enter your body, filling and nourishing the Kidneys, hydrating every cell in your body.

Small Circle

The Small Circle is the first part of Turning and Winding the Belt Vessel and is practiced to initiate movement in the Belt Vessel and Gate of Life. Practice this exercise to warm up before continuing on to the Large Circle. When turning the Small Circle, the focus on the waist remains closer to the front of the body and the lower dantian.

1 **Start in the beginning posture. You may want to step out just a bit, widening the stance to give yourself enough room to move during this exercise. Shift your weight to the right leg so that the knees are in alignment with the hips and shoulders, all stacked one above the other. Turn your torso so that the front centerline of the chest faces about 45 degrees to the right. Lift the hands by bending at the elbows and let the hands rest on an imaginary surface that is waist high, palms down. Prepare to inhale. Most of your awareness should be on the waist area. Visualize yourself standing in a pool of water that is waist deep. Your hands are resting on the surface of the water. Keep the body relaxed. The shoulders are soft and dropped; avoid tensing the neck and shoulders. The wrists are relaxed.**

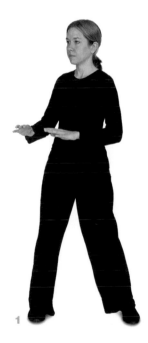

1

(continued)

Small Circle *(continued)*

2 Begin by shifting your weight to the left leg. Do this by pulling from the left leg instead of pushing from the right leg. This helps to smooth out the transition and avoids bobbing up and down. Once your weight is on the left leg, make sure your ankles, knees, hips, and shoulders are all in good alignment, one over the other. Then turn the torso until it is facing 45 degrees to the left. You will keep the knees facing forward and there will be a crease in the hips. The hands will also turn to the left as a result of turning the torso. Once your hands begin to travel forward and along the circle's edge toward the left, begin to inhale. The hands are moving away from the lower dantian and are making the far edge of a circle that lies horizontally in front of you. The inhalation matches the movement so that you are inhaling as your hands move away from the body. The purpose of this qigong is to turn the Belt Vessel, so let your awareness settle on the area of your waist, the lower dantian, and the Ming Men. As you turn, you should be reaching for the Belt Vessel to assist in turning it in the next step. This step is also for tonifying: Visualize your hands gathering water and healthy Kidney qi.

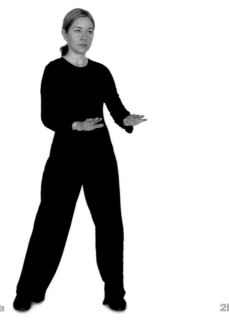

2a

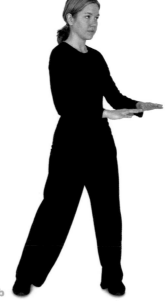

2b

3 Once your torso is facing 45 degrees to the left and you've finished inhaling, it's time to retract, or return. Begin to exhale and shift your weight onto the right leg by pulling from the right leg instead of pushing from the left. As your body shifts sides, the hands turn the palms toward the lower dantian and retract closer to the belly. The movement finishes with the hands still facing the lower dantian, weight on the right leg, and the torso facing the right. This final position is the same as the beginning of step 1 except the palms are still facing the lower dantian and not resting on the surface of the water. In the previous step, you connected to and stretched the Belt Vessel; now turn it with your mind and allow the Water qi you've collected with your hands to enter the lower dantian and left Kidney. A simple way to remember the proper sequence and to coordinate the movements is *shift and turn*: First shift your weight and then turn the body. After a few repetitions, try to smooth out the shifting and turning so that a smooth circle is created and the rhythm is seamless.

Repeat steps 2 and 3 for at least nine repetitions in a counterclockwise motion (expanding from right to left, contracting from left to right). Then proceed to the transition.

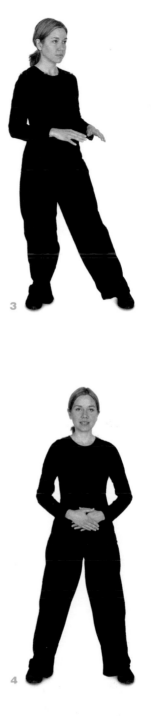

4 This step repeats the motions but in a clockwise circle. Perform the transition movement to switch sides as follows: Once you've finished the last repetition, you should be on the right leg with the palms facing your lower dantian. Return your weight to the left leg and have the torso face 45 degrees to the left. The hands come out onto the surface of the water you're standing in. You are now ready to repeat the circular motions in a clockwise manner. During the transition, there is no particular breath, and the mind returns to a neutral or center point until you're ready to begin the next movement.

(continued)

Small Circle *(continued)*

5 After completing the transition, your weight is on the left leg and the torso is facing 45 degrees to the left. The next step is identical to step 2 but in a clockwise manner. Begin to inhale and expand the arms to trace the top side of the circle from left to right. As soon as you begin to inhale, begin shifting the weight from left to right. The hands will drift out and turn when the torso turns to the right. Once your hands begin to travel forward and along the edge of the circle toward the right, begin to inhale. The inhalation matches the movement so that you are inhaling as your hands move away from the body and the torso turns. Your awareness should be on the Belt Vessel connecting the hands to the qi that flows along the waist, guiding it to turn and stretch with the movement of the body.

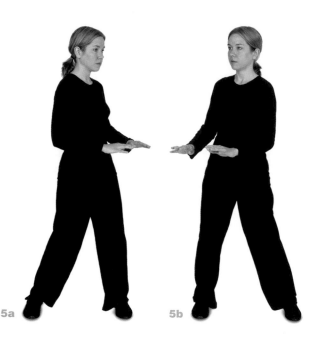

5a   5b

6 Perform step 3 in the opposite direction. Repeat steps 5 and 6 for at least nine repetitions in a clockwise motion (expanding from left to right, contracting from right to left). Then proceed to the Large Circle.

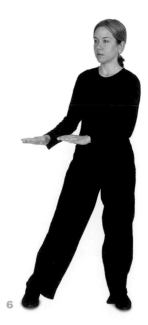

6

Large Circle

The Large Circle is similar to the Small Circle, only the arms travel beyond the front of the torso all the way around to the back. The extra extension of the arms and eyes allows for a deeper stretch of the Belt Vessel, providing greater movement of qi.

1 **After completing the Small Circle, return to the beginning posture as described in step 1 of the Small Circle so that your weight is on the right leg and your body is turned 45 degrees to the right. Bring the hands to rest on the surface of the water. As you begin to inhale, let the hands travel outward, tracing the circle counterclockwise. As your body turns to the left, shift your weight onto the left leg, observing the rules of structure (knees above the ankles, hips above the knees, shoulders in alignment with the hips). Turn the body so that the hands travel all the way around the body to rest on the waist in the back. Turn your head so that the eyes are looking behind you. Both palms should be facing and resting on the waist. This movement is supported by inhaling. The inhalation matches the movement beginning when the hands are on the right and ending when the hands are on the waist. As with the previous circle, your awareness should be on moving the Belt Vessel, but this time the hands are connecting with the Belt Vessel at its source on the Ming Men and turning it widely from one side to the other. This step is also for tonifying; therefore, collect healthy Water qi to nourish the Kidneys and fill the lower dantian.**

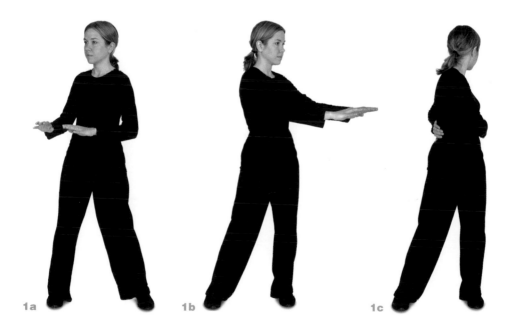

1a   1b   1c

(continued)

Large Circle *(continued)*

2 The next step is to return to facing forward and return your weight onto the right leg. To do this, begin the motion from the right hip, shifting your weight back onto the right leg. Turn the torso so that it faces 45 degrees to the right. This will naturally slide the hands along the waist back toward the front. End with your hands facing the lower dantian parallel with the midline of the body. This movement is supported by exhaling. The exhalation matches the movement beginning when the hands are on the waist and ending when the hands are on the lower dantian. Having connected to the Belt Vessel, assist the turning of its qi with your hands, breath, and mind. If using the exercise for tonifying, then allow the Water qi you collected to be stored in the Kidneys and to fill the lower dantian.

Repeat steps 1 and 2 for at least nine repetitions in a counterclockwise motion (expanding from right to left, contracting from left to right), then transition by keeping your hands on the lower dantian, shifting your weight onto the left leg, and turning the torso so that it faces 45 degrees to the left. During the transition, there is no particular breath, and the mind returns to a neutral or center point until ready to begin the next movement.

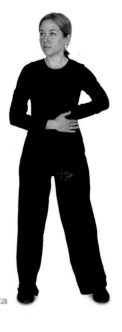

2a

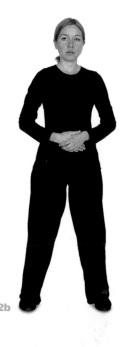

2b

3 From the end of the transition point, let the hands extend so that they are resting on the surface of the water again. Your body should be facing 45 degrees to the left. Begin by shifting your weight to the right leg. As you move your weight onto the right leg, let the hands expand straight out in front so that they can begin to trace the top part of the circle clockwise. Once your body is in alignment on the right, turn the torso. This will automatically move the hands along the edge of the circle. Turn as far as you can, bringing the palms to rest on the waist and turning the head so that you can look straight behind you. Breath should be one long inhalation from the beginning of the movement on the left all the way until your eyes are looking behind you. Allow the body to relax as it turns and let the mind settle on the Belt Vessel after your hands rest on your waist.

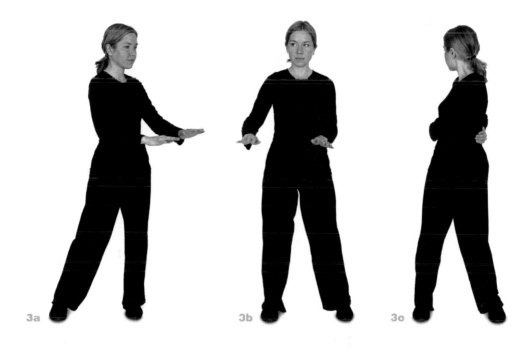

3a 3b 3o

(continued)

Large Circle *(continued)*

4 The next step is to contract and return to face the left. Simply shift your weight onto the left leg as in step 2 and begin to turn the torso toward the left. The hands will naturally follow. End with the body weight on the left leg and the torso 45 degrees to the left, palms down on the surface of the water. The breath matches the movement, exhaling from the back all the way to the front. Your awareness should be on turning the Belt Vessel and relaxing. Repeat steps 3 and 4 for at least nine repetitions in a clockwise motion (expanding from left to right, contracting from right to left).

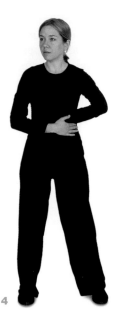

5 Once you've completed the last repetition, return to face forward with the palms of both hands resting on the lower dantian. Take three deep breaths, allowing the qi to settle into the lower dantian.

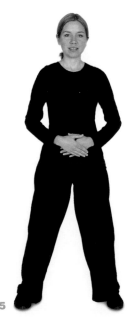

Turning and Winding the Belt Vessel

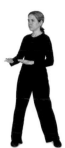 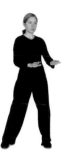 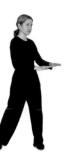 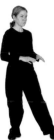 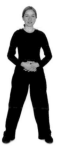

Page 117   Page 118   Page 118   Page 119   Page 119

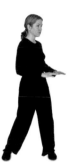 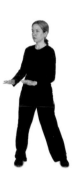 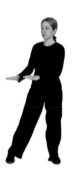 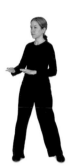 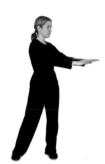

Page 120   Page 120   Page 120   Page 121   Page 121

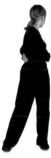 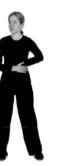 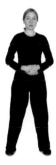 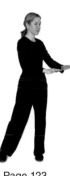 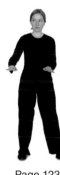

Page 121   Page 122   Page 122   Page 123   Page 123

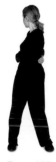 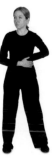 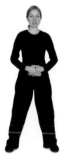

Page 123   Page 124   Page 124

Chapter 9

Qigong for Relaxation

Now that your organs and meridians are thoroughly cleansed and reenergized, it's time to return your thoughts and awareness to your center (Taiji Pole) and settle the qi before proceeding with the rest of the day's activities. This section corresponds to the cool-down phase of a complete qigong routine. If you have performed all the sections from chapter 6 to chapter 8, these next three exercises are perfect for slowing down and rooting your qi to the lower dantian.

In chapter 5, we described many of the benefits of rooting qi into the lower dantian. We learned that the mind leads the qi, which leads the jing. For the entire qigong routine, we have used our mind to direct qi to specific areas of the body to promote health and healing. This section is directed at stabilizing the connection between the mind and the body without a particular focused intention. Since the body is already relaxed, most of our work is done. Finishing with the mind allows us to retain the ability to focus and stay calm for longer periods of time and through chaotic or stressful situations. When the mind is unsettled, our thoughts are random, frantic, and easily distracted by small details. Attention to this section of the qigong routine promotes tranquility, clarity, and peace.

Outside of the qigong practice, there are many times when we wish we had a natural remedy for stressful situations, a little something we could do to help restore feelings of peace and serenity. Qigong offers many solutions to stress, from hour-long workouts to 15-minute meditations, but the following three exercises are quick and to-the-point qigong movements that promote instant relaxation. They are easy to do and require only a few minutes of time. They can be done alone anytime you need to freshen up or as a conclusion to a longer qigong workout. Although they are quite simple, their effectiveness is immediate.

Swimming Dragon

Sliding through the water by waving its tail left and right, the Swimming Dragon restores tranquility by rooting the mind in the lower dantian. The rhythmic side-to-side motion of the body and the deep breathing also relax the waist and hips, promoting deep internal circulation of Blood and qi. The Swimming Dragon is a good way to center your awareness and build qi in the lower dantian. It can be considered a tonification exercise because it brings in qi to nourish the Kidneys. The actual movement of this qigong is of gathering qi into the lower dantian by extending the hands out to the sides and scooping water into the belly. Throughout this qigong, see yourself gliding through gentle waters, gathering peacefulness and finding harmony in your center.

1 Start in the beginning posture. Bring both hands to rest over the lower dantian with the palms facing the belly. Begin by turning your body to the right so that the torso faces 45 degrees to the right. At the same time, the right hand slides across the belly, slowly reaching out 45 degrees to the back. Once the right hand is extended, begin to turn the hips and torso toward the left. This will bring the right hand around in a circular motion; be sure to keep it at waist height as you bring the palm around to face the belly. The inhalation begins with the right hand in the back corner and ends when the right hand is in front of the midline of the body with the palm facing the belly again. As your hand glides through the water, visualize qi being collected into your hand as if you were filling a large bowl.

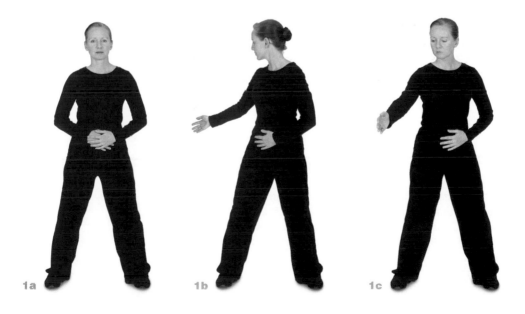

1a   1b   1c

(continued)

Swimming Dragon *(continued)*

2 As the right palm begins to turn and face the belly, complete the circle by bringing the palm closer to the body and finally resting on the lower dantian. Simultaneously, as the right hand begins to approach the belly, the left hand reaches out 45 degrees to the rear left-hand corner, preparing to scoop from the left side. Exhale as the right palm approaches the belly and the left hand reaches out. Visualize the qi gathered in the right hand, soaking into and being stored in the lower dantian.

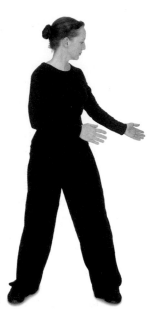

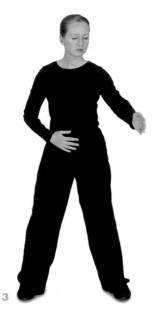

3 With the right hand facing the belly and the left hand extended, you're ready to scoop from the left side. Begin to turn the hips and torso toward the right, naturally bringing the left hand around in a scooping motion. Inhale while gathering qi from the left side. Visualize your left hand scooping in healthy, nourishing qi in the form of water and bringing it closer to the lower dantian. This is a repetition of the same action from the right side but now on the left side.

4 The left hand is now ready to approach the lower dantian, so complete the circle by bringing the left palm to rest on the lower belly. At the same time, the right hand is sliding out to the to begin the next repetition. Exhale as the right hand reaches toward the back. Visualize the gathered qi being absorbed and stored in the lower dantian.

Repeat the scooping and storing motion on both sides of the body, alternating left and right for a count of 12 repetitions to each side. End with the left hand on top of the right hand, both resting on the lower dantian.

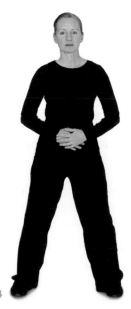

Rising Lotus Facial Rejuvenation

Among the many benefits of practicing qigong is the youthful glow of radiant health. Our skin and appearance can change noticeably with even just one session of qigong. By removing any turbid qi that surrounds our body and creating a peaceful mental state, the natural glow of our inner being is free to shine through, reflecting our inner radiance. This simple qigong exercise replaces expensive creams, offering an organic and eco-friendly option that never runs out. During the Rising Lotus Facial Rejuvenation qigong, we use qi to create an impeccable facial cream charged with as many ingredients as we wish. No need to worry about clashing fragrances or allergic reactions—this cream is Divine! With repeated use, your skin will be rejuvenated, drawing compliments and leaving people to wonder just what your secret is.

Throughout this exercise, relax and find the joy in cherishing the beautiful things life has to offer. Raise your thoughts and vibration as high as possible by surrounding yourself with as many healing and nourishing thoughts as possible. Imbue the cream with all these intentions and then enjoy the immediate results! As part of a larger qigong routine, you would normally repeat this qigong three times; however, you may repeat these steps as many times as you like.

1 **Start in the beginning posture, but be sure to relax the body and let this qigong be natural. There are no exact rules to follow, but the visualization process in this qigong is important. Bring your palms in front of your torso in the same manner as in shaping a ball of dough—one palm up and one palm down, fingers pointing in opposite directions. Let the hands face each other for a few breaths without moving. Then begin to move them so that you're creating an energy ball between the palms. Breathe naturally during this qigong; no need to focus on inhaling or exhaling. Use your intention to condense qi between the palms and to create the cream. As the qi begins to condense between your palms, give the cream as many characteristics as possible. Feel its weight (heavy or light), consistency (thick or silky), and temperature (warm or cold); give it a color and a fragrance; add healing herbs to it or other ingredients you think will benefit your skin. This cream can become anything you want, so take as much time as you like to ensure that the cream is everything you want it to be.**

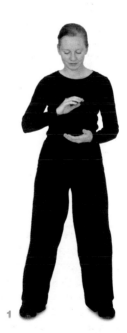

1

(continued)

Rising Lotus Facial Rejuvenation *(continued)*

2 Once you've created the cream, turn the palms so that the fingers point up. You will be holding the ball of cream in front of you, the hands acting as a pedestal. Exhale in preparation for the next step. Use your awareness to hold the cream in your hands, making sure you don't drop the cream or lose the visualization. See the cream resting in your palms, waiting to be spread over your skin.

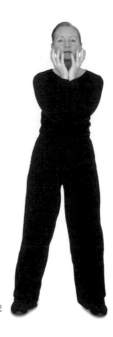

2

3 Begin to bring the hands closer to the chin, fingers pointing up toward the hairline as if they were holding a bowl. Dip your chin into the lotus that holds the cream and allow your fingers and palms to slide up the front of your face all the way to the hairline. Inhale for the length of time it takes to bring the hands up to the chin and across your face up to the hairline. This part of the qigong is spreading the cream over your face, so feel all the qualities you charged your cream with now being absorbed by your skin, instantly changing the structure of your complexion.

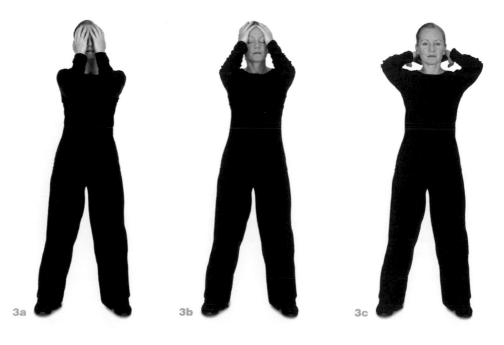

3a   3b   3c

4 Once your fingers reach the hairline, begin to exhale and scoop your fingers as if you were pulling off something from your head and body. Briefly shake out your hands to release any "sludge" you pulled off. Then, bring your hands back to the front to form another energy ball. The cream has all been spread on the face, so now it's time to create some more. Bring your awareness back between the palms and begin the next energy ball. You may feel some sludge on your palms after spreading the cream, so take some time to purify the cream and recharge it with all the qualities you want it to have.

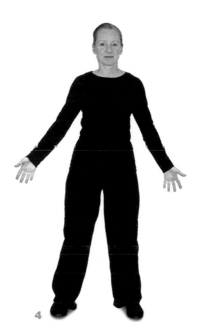

4

Ten Dragons Running Through the Forest

This is a thoroughly tested and proven method for clearing head fog, stressful thoughts, and even headaches! As the name implies, 10 dragons will be running through the forest, otherwise known as your hair. The dragons are represented by each of your fingers. A lot of qi is created and accumulated by the activity of our mind, and as the dragons meander and weave their way forward, they pull away anything that no longer serves your highest good, leaving behind a clear trail of peace and tranquility. As part of a larger qigong routine, you would normally repeat this qigong three times. However, you may repeat these steps as many times as you like.

1 **Start in the beginning posture; however, this is a simple qigong so be sure to be comfortable and relaxed. Bring your fingers up to the hairline at the forehead with all the fingertips touching the head lightly. Using light pressure, move the fingers from the hairline toward the back of the head, ending just at the bottom of the occiput. Your fingers will trace a semicircle following the two sides of your head above the ears and down to the nape of the neck. Inhale as the hands move from the hairline all the way until they stop at the occiput. Visualize the dragons eating away any tension that has accumulated at the head and clearing away any turbid qi.**

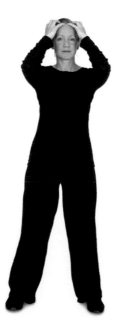

1a

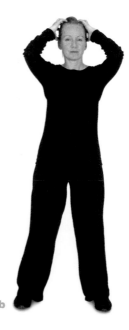

1b

2 In the previous step, the hands stopped at the occiput. This next step involves pulling away the turbid qi from the head and discarding it. Simply close your fingers at the occiput as if you were grabbing a fist full of sticky substance. Pull it away from the head and flick your hands as if you were clearing the stickiness off your hands. Support the release of any turbid qi by exhaling during this step. Visualize turbid qi being pulled away from the body in the hands and discarded into the Earth to be transformed and purified.

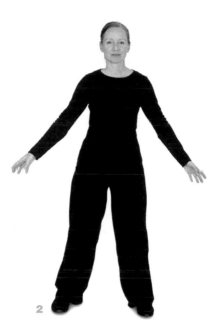

2

This completes a full qigong routine from opening to cooling down. To finish and close your practice time, do three Pulling Down Heavens as described in chapter 5 under the section on closing. Visualize the three columns of light: white in the center, silver down the front, and gold down the back. Allow yourself to take three long breaths upon finishing the Pulling Down Heavens; during these breaths, allow the mind to settle in the center and clear your thoughts. There should be no focused intention other than breathing and relaxing. When you're ready, you can then move on to the next activity of the day.

Now that you've practiced a full qigong routine from start to finish, you should feel energized, relaxed, and centered. Many people say that practicing qigong produces feelings of cold, warmth, tingling, wind, chills, and vibrations in the body during and after practice. In most cases, this is nothing to worry about. If the symptoms persist for more than a few days or for more than six hours after you finished practicing, then you may want to consult an experienced qigong practitioner for advice.

Upon initiating a qigong practice, you may also notice a shift in your eating, sleeping, or overall energy patterns. Each person is different, so these shifts can mean increased eating, sleeping, or energy, but there can also be a temporary dip. In both cases, any sharp differences will be quickly worked through and a stable pattern should develop. These changes are due to energy blocks being released and the meridians opening up. Some shifts can be over in just a few minutes, whereas other shifts may take a few weeks. In any case, if you are practicing without a teacher, know that most of these changes are normal. If in doubt, contact a qualified instructor.

If it's your first time practicing qigong, you may still have many questions about how to practice particular moves or routines. Don't let these questions get in the way of your practice. It's not important to be precise at this point—what is important is getting started, creating a habit of doing movement, and taking time for yourself.

For additional information, you may consult the author at www.therisinglotus.com or reputable organizations such as the following:

► National Qigong Association (www.nqa.org)

► Qigong Institute (www.qigonginstitute.org)

► International Institute of Medical Qigong (www.medicalqigong.org)

Appendix:
History of Qigong

It is important to note that dates are approximate since the accuracy of history is under current examination by Chinese Historians and Scholars. In addition, different sources may attribute extremely early works to different sources. This interpretation is based on the more traditional versions of the development of Chinese Medicine, Qigong, and the Dynasties.

3 Sovereigns 5 Emperors X-2070 BCE[1]	Xia Dynasty 2070-1600 BCE	Shang Dynasty 1600-1045 BCE	Western Zhou Dynasty 1045-771 BCE	Spring & Autumn Period 772-476 BCE	Warring States Period 403-221 BCE	Qin & Han Dynasty 220BCE-221CE
Emperor *Fú Xu* c. 2953-2838 Begins using the trigrams (...of the I Ching)	**Shamans** began the use of pyromancy via oracle bones. Few artifacts have been found.	**Birth of Qigong** First developments into a more systematic practice		**Lao Tzu** is said to have lived during this time. Exact date is unknown	c. 300 **Zhuang Zi** described relationship between health and breath in his book *Nan Hua Zhen Jing*, aka *The Chuang Tzu.*	*Nan Jing Classic on Disorders* by Bian Chiueh
	Yi Jing First written record of the Yi Jing is traditionally credited to this period.	**Birth of Acupuncture** First use of stones to stimulate acupuncture points		**Dao De Jing** was written by Lao Tzu describing advanced breathing techniques.[2]	**Huang Di Nei Jing** *Yellow Emperors Inner Classic* was written.	**Jin Gui Yao Lue** *Prescriptions from the Golden Chamber* by Chang Chung-Gieh
		Proliferation of **oracle bones** bearing information on qi cultivation.[3] Most artifacts found are from this period.		**Buddha** Siddhartha Gautama lives c. 563-483	**Zhuang Zi** lives c. 370-290	**Hua Tuo** lives and creates **Wuqinxi (5 Animal Frolic).**
				Confucius lives c. 551-479	The term **Dao Yin** was adopted to describe the various qigong exercises.	**Mawangdui** (Dao Yin Tu) silk text was created.
					Buddhism arrives in China but is suppressed and undocumented.	c.58 CE Official acceptance of Buddhism having migrated from India to China with translation of *Sutra of 42 Chapters* into Chinese
					c. 221 The Great Wall of China is built.	Birth of **Chan Buddhism**, "father" of Zen Buddhism

Daoists and Shamans during the early Dynasties focused on developing a deep understanding of the interaction and cycles of the energies of Heaven, Man and Earth – The Three Treasures. The I Ching went through several stages of development.

Throughout this period, qigong was predominantly used by Daoists seeking to live in harmony with nature. Non-Daoists began to take notice as incredible health accomplishments are obtained through the manipulation of qi.

Due to the success of treating health conditions by practicing and understanding qi, physicians and scholars actively began studying, transcribing, and documenting their knowledge.

[1] Encyclopedia of Taoism by Fabrizio Pregadio. The Eight Pieces of Brocade, 1988, 1992, by Dr. Yang Jwing-Ming
[2] Chinese Qigong Illustrated, 1995, by Yu Gongbao. Wikipedia: http://en.wikipedia.org/wiki/Dynasties_in_Chinese_history
[3] Wikipedia: http://en.wikipedia.org/wiki/Oracle_bone

Six Dynasties: 3 Kingdoms, Western and Eastern Jin, Northern and Southern Dynasties 220 CE-589 CE	Sui & Tang Dynasties 581-907 CE	Northern & Southern Song Dynasties 960-1279 CE	Yuan Dynasty 1279-1368 CE / Ming Dynasty 1368-1644 CE	Qing Dynasty 1644-1911 CE	Republic of China 1911-today / People's Republic of China 1949-today
Religious Qigong is born as Buddhism (aimed at reaching Buddhahood) blends with previous qigong practices. This type of qigong was secret and only taught in temples.	c.610 **Zhu Bing Yun Hou Lun** *Thesis on the Origins and Symptoms of Various Diseases* was written by Chao YuanFang.	c. 12th century **Chang San-Feng** creates **Tai Qi Chuan.** Internal Elixir (NeiDan) emerges.	c.1644-1911 **BaGuaZhang** emerges and is attributed to **Dong Hai-Chuan.**	**Chen, Yang, Wu, and Sun** **Tai chi Chuan** lineages emerge.	China's borders begin to open, and the qigong and martial arts reach world access. The effect is bilateral in that the art is learned by non-Chinese in its purity but later changed, adapted, and transformed according to local and cultural influences.
c.34-156 **Zhang DaoLing** established the 5 Pecks of Rice – ZhengYi Tradition.	c. 652 **Beiji Qianjin** Yaofang *Thousand Gold Prescriptions* was written by Sun SiMiao.	c.1127-1279 **Eight Pieces of Brocade** was created by **Marshal Yeuh Fei.**	By this period Tai Chi and Qigong have spread throughout China and begin evolving into unique family styles or systems based on local and personal application.	Proliferation of qigong and martial arts styles	Cigong accelerates into global view.
Tibetan Buddhism arrives in China. **Ge Hong** lives c. 283-343.	Martial Qigong expands greatly due to Da Mo's influence at the Shaolin Temple giving rise to the **Five Kung Fu Styles:** Tiger, Leopard, Dragon, Crane & Snake.	**Marshal Yeuh Fei** creates **Xing Yi Chuan.**	The America's are "discovered" by Christopher Columbus in 1492.		**Daoist Five Qigong** is created.
c.502-557 **Da Mo** (Indian Prince and Buddhist monk) settles in the Shaolin temple giving birth to **martial qigong.** Author of **Yi Jin Jing** (Muscle/Tendon Changing Classic) and **Xi Sui Jing** (Brain Marrow Washing Classic)	Lu DongBin Born c. 638 **External Elixir Qigong (Wei Dan)**				Religious Qigong and meditative practices remain obscure and private following the tradition of being passed on by teacher to student.

Glossary

axilla—The hollow beneath the arm; armpit.

breath—Another term for qi; the air we breathe.

Bubbling Well—English name for the acupuncture point Kidney 1 (Yong Quan), located on the bottom of the foot and through which qi flows up from the Earth.

Conception Vessel—One of the eight Extraordinary Vessels. (Vessels are similar to meridians.) The Conception Vessel runs along the front midline of the body from the perineum up to the mouth, where it connects to the Governing Vessel. The conception vessel distributes yin qi throughout the body and is known as the sea of yin.

dantian—Literally translates as "elixir field" and can be interpreted as an energy field. There are three dantian in the body: the pelvic region (lower dantian), the center of the chest (middle dantian), and the head (upper dantian). The dantian are one of the correlations of the Three Treasures.

Five Elements Theory—a theory of energetic balance between the energies of water, wood, fire, earth and metal. The original term in Chinese is *WuXing* and is translated as the "5 Phases". *WuXing* is used to describes the interaction of the 5 elements throughout the myriad manifestations of the universe.

Water—one of the five elements; relates to the Kidneys. See page 33-34.

Wood—one of the five elements; relates to Liver. See page 33-34.

Fire—one of the five elements; relates to the Heart. See page 33-34.

Earth—one of the five elements; relates to the Spleen. See page 33-34.

Metal—one of the five elements; relates to the Lungs. See page 33-34.

Gate of Life (Ming Men)—Located at the acupuncture point known as GV 4 on the lower back, just above the sacrum, it is one of the major energy points along the Governing Vessel.

Governing Vessel—One of the eight Extraordinary Vessels. (Vessels are similar to meridians.) The Governing Vessel runs along the rear midline of the body over the spine from the sacrum and into the mouth, where it connects to the Conception Vessel. The Governing Vessel distributes yang qi throughout the body and is known as the sea of yang.

intention—The way we direct our mind or thoughts while practicing qigong; sometimes can be interpreted as will or purpose.

jing—Essence; vital substance.

meridians—The body's channels or rivers through which qi is distributed throughout the body.

occiput—The lower back part of the head where the skull meets the cervical vertebrae.

perineum—The area between the anus and the genitals.

posture—The alignment of bones and joints; otherwise known as physical structure.

qi—Energy, life force, or breath.

qigong—Energy cultivation; a collection of meditations and movements to support martial, medical (health), or spiritual training.

medical qigong—Qigong movements practiced in order to elicit healing for a specific health condition.

medical qigong therapy—One of the branches of traditional Chinese medicine; a healing modality in which a therapist transmits qi to a patient for the purpose of improving health.

shen—Spirit; also related to the mind.

Taiji Pole—Column of qi that runs between the top of the head and the perineum.

Three Treasures—Describes several three-tiered relationships, including Heaven, Man, and Earth, or jing, qi, and shen.

yang—Quality of energy that is hard, inflexible, male, and so on.

yin—Quality of energy that is soft, yielding, feminine, and so on.

wei qi field—Literally translates as "external energy;" a qi (energy) bubble that surrounds the body.

WuXing—the five phases. See Five Elements Theory.

Resources

Organizations

National Qigong Association (www.nqa.org)
Qigong Institute (www.qigonginstitute.org)
International Institute of Medical Qigong (www.medicalqigong.com)

Publications

The Web That Has No Weaver by Ted Kaptchuk
The Way of Qigong by Ken Cohen
Chinese Medical Qigong by Tianjin Liu, OMD and Kevin Chen, PhD
Chinese Medical Qigong Therapy (Vol. 1-5) by Prof. Jerry Alan Johnson

DVDs

Chi Kung: The Healing Workout by Jerry Alan Johnson
Qigong Beginning Practice by Francesco Garripoli

About the Author

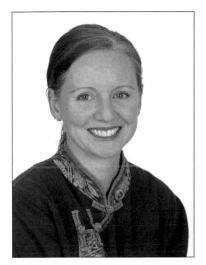

Christina J. Barea is an ordained Daoist priest who holds a master's degree in medical qigong (MMQ) from the International Institute of Medical Qigong (IIMQ), where she studied with internationally recognized founders Dr. Jerry Alan Johnson and Dr. Bernard Shannon. She is a certified level III qigong instructor through the National Qigong Association and has taught at the University of East-West Medicine. She is also a member of the National Qigong Association's board of directors.

Barea was born and raised in Puerto Rico and is fluent in English, Spanish, and Italian. She currently resides in Atlanta, Georgia and enjoys spending time in nature, playing the Native American flute, and exploring other cultures.

Barea is also proud to be collaborating with Sheri Gilburth (middle) and Essud Fungcap (right) who graciously donated their time to model for this book. Sheri Gilburth is a gifted healer who specializes in energetic therapy through various modalities such as Reiki, Pranic Healing, Hypnotherapy, Craniosacral Therapy, and Shamanism. Essud Fungcap is a talented mind-body instructor who guides people into radiant health with an eclectic blend of yoga, tai chi, and qigong. Sheri, Essud, and Christina are founding members of Heart Center Therapy in Atlanta, Georgia where they share their talents to promote whole-body health. Please visit www.heartcentertherapy.com for more information.

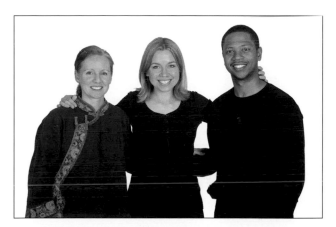

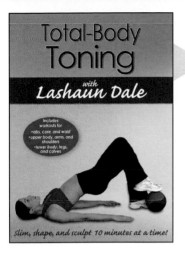
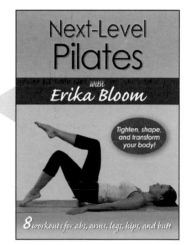
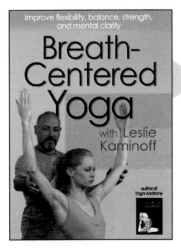

ANATOMY SERIES

Each book in the *Anatomy Series* provides detailed, full-color anatomical illustrations of the muscles in action and step-by-step instructions that detail perfect technique and form for each pose, exercise, movement, stretch, and stroke.

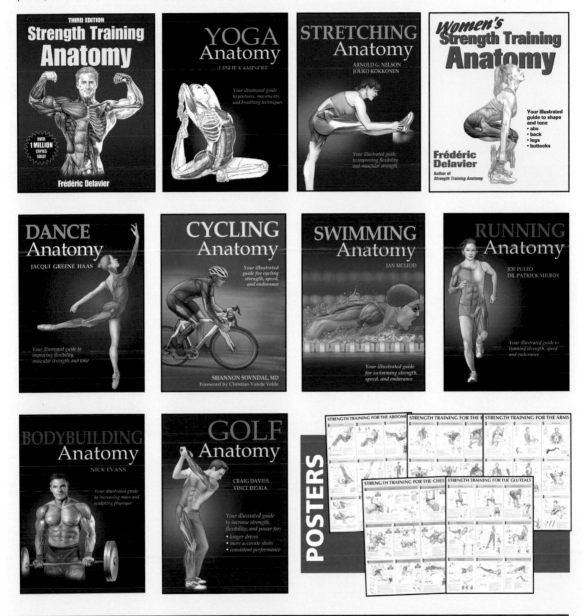

To place your order, U.S. customers call TOLL FREE **1-800-747-4457**
In Canada call 1-800-465-7301 • In Europe call +44 (0) 113 255 5665 • In Australia call 08 8372 0999
In New Zealand call 0800 222 062 • or visit **www.HumanKinetics.com/Anatomy**

HUMAN KINETICS
The Premier Publisher for Sports & Fitness
P.O. Box 5076, Champaign, IL 61825-5076

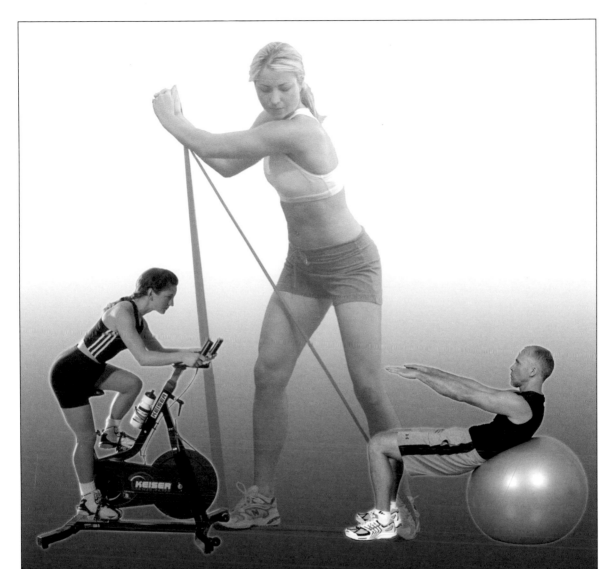

You'll find other outstanding fitness resources at

www.HumanKinetics.com/fitnessandhealth

In the U.S. call 1-800-747-4457

Australia 08 8372 0999 • Canada 1-800-465-7301
Europe +44 (0) 113 255 5665 • New Zealand 0800 222 062

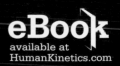